With compliments

Knoll AG

BASF Pharma

knoll

Springer

Berlin
Heidelberg
New York
Barcelona
Budapest
Hong Kong
London
Mailand
Paris
Santa Clara
Singapore
Tokyo

G. Abatangelo   L. Donati
W. Vanscheidt   (Eds.)

Proteolysis in Wound Repair

With Contributions by
G. Abatangelo, P. Altmeyer, V. Bizot-Foulon, L. Cardarelli,
R. Cortivo, J. M. Davidson, M. De Simone, C. el Gammal,
J. F. Hansbrough, W. Hansbrough, W. Hornebeck,
G. Lafranco, A. Meddahi, J. R. Mekkes, G. Murphy,
M. Nano, W. C. Parks, B. Pellat, R. Popp, M. Radice,
E. Ricci, M. Schäfer, W. Westerhof, J. E. Zeegelaar

With 30 Colored Figures

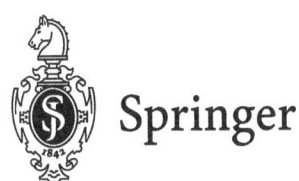 Springer

G. Abatangelo
Institute of Histology
Faculty of Medicine
University of Padua
Italy

L. Donati
Institute of Plastic Surgery
Milan
Italy

W. Vanscheidt
Universitäts-Hautklinik
Hauptstr. 7
79104 Freiburg i.Br.

Springer-Verlag GmbH & Co. KG
Science Communication
Editing Dept. for Medicine
Dr. B. Fruhstorfer
U. Hilpert, D. Berger, K. Kupfer, Dr. Ch. Leist,
Dr. N. Mosler, Heidelberg

Cover: View of the Palazzo della Ragione and Piazza delle Erbe

ISBN-13:978-3-540-60815-8   e-ISBN-13:978-3-642-61130-8
DOI: 10.1007/978-3-642-61130-8

Layout and Production Supervision: W. Bischoff, Heidelberg
Cover Design: W. Bischoff, Heidelberg
Typesetting, Reproduction of Figures, Printing and

SPIN 10501529 16 / 3134 – 5 4 3 2 1 0 – Printed on acid-free paper

Contents

G. Abatangelo
Institute of Histology, Faculty of Medicine,
University of Padua, Italy

P. Altmeyer
Department of Dermatology, Ruhr University of Bochum,
Germany

V. Bizot-Foulon
Laboratory of Biochemistry, Faculty of Dental Surgery,
University René Descartes-Paris V, Montrouge, France

L. Cardarelli
Institute of Histology, Faculty of Medicine,
University of Padua, Italy

R. Cortivo
Institute of Histology, Faculty of Medicine,
University of Padua, Italy

J. M. Davidson
Department of Pathology, Vanderbilt University,
Nashville, TN, USA

M. De Simone
Department of Clinical Pathophysiology
and Geriatric Surgery, University of Turin, Italy

L. Donati
Institute of Plastic Surgery, University of Milan, Italy

C. el Gammal
Department of Dermatology, Ruhr University of Bochum,
Germany

S. el Gammal
Department of Dermatology, Ruhr University of Bochum,
Germany

J. F. Hansbrough
Department of Surgery, University of California,
San Diego Medical Center, San Diego, CA, USA

W. Hansbrough
Department of Surgery, University of California,
San Diego Medical Center, San Diego, CA, USA

W. Hornebeck
Laboratory of Biochemistry, Faculty of Dental Surgery,
University René Descartes-Paris V, Montrouge, France
and Laboratory CRRET, University of Paris XII, Créteil, France

G. Lanfranco
Departments of Clinical Pathophysiology
and Geriatric Surgery, University of Turin, Italy

A. Meddahi
Laboratory CRRET, University of Paris XII, Créteil, France

J. R. Mekkes
Department of Dermatology, Academic Medical Center,
Amsterdam, The Netherlands

G. Murphy
Strangeways Research Laboratory, Cambridge,
United Kingdom

M. Nano
Departments of Clinical Pathophysiology
and Geriatric Surgery, University of Turin, Italy

W. C. Parks
Division of Dermatology, Jewish Hospital, Washington
University School of Medicine, St. Louis, MO, USA

B. Pellat
Laboratory of Biochemistry, Faculty of Dental Surgery,
University René Descartes-Paris V, Montrouge, France

R. Popp
Clinical Research Department, Knoll AG, Ludwigshafen,
Germany

M. Radice
Institute of Histology, Faculty of Medicine,
University of Padua, Italy

E. Ricci
Departments of Clinical Pathophysiology
and Geriatric Surgery, University of Turin, Italy

M. Schäfer
Technical Development Department ZET/SZ, BASF AG,
Ludwigshafen, Germany

W. Westerhof
Department of Dermatology, Academic Medical Center,
Amsterdam, The Netherlands

J. E. Zeegelaar
Department of Dermatology, Academic Medical Center,
Amsterdam, The Netherlands

Preface

Extracellular matrix (ECM) turnover is a widespread but incompletely understood process. Many studies have been conducted with the aim of discovering the general mechanisms which produce and maintain the ECM in tissues. Wound repair in animals has always been a suitable "tool" for exploring these mechanisms. In such a pathologic event, the different components of the healing system can be readily observed since they are exaggerated. It has now become clear that the regulation of protease/inhibitor activity is one of the most important steps in maintaining the integrity of ECM in the normal as well as in the pathologic state. As far as the repair process is concerned, a failure in such regulation may result in abnormal wound healing ranging from nonhealing wounds to hypertrophic scarring.

Experimental findings have been directly applied in clinical practice. For example, the importance of débridement in normal and especially in poorly healing wounds has become much clearer in the recent past. Different methods have been proposed to obtain an optimal wound bed in order to perform skin transplantation.

Both mechanical and physical débridement procedures undoubtedly offer some advantages and are essential when extensive third degree burns have to be treated. On the other hand, pain, excessive blood loss, and overall broad and indiscriminate débridement are common negative side effects. Thus, many enzymic formulations have been proposed and used in practice by clinicians all over the world. From different studies enzymatic débridement appears to have the potential of generating a clean wound bed and a gentle eschar removal. Preparations involving natural healing proteinases such as collagenases have been shown to release the eschar without affecting the underneath viable granulation tissue.

The symposium "Proteolysis in Wound Healing" took place during the 5th Annual Meeting of the European Tissue Repair Society, held in Padua from August 30 until September 2, 1995. Lectures on the important subject of enzymatic débridement were held, and this book reports on some of the scientific concepts presented there.

My personal impression is that there have been many improvements in molecular biology and in clinical research during the last few years. These new experimental findings and therapeutic approaches will certainly be of tremendous help to those clinicians who are dealing with abnormal tissue repair problems.

Giovanni Abatangelo, MD, PhD
President of the Organizing Committee
of the 5th Annual Meeting
of the European Tissue Repair Society
President of the ETRS

It is a great honor to introduce this volume which reports on the experience of a select group of researchers and of clinicians. Both are vital to our understanding, of tissue repair, for it has recently become clear that it is mandatory to fill the gap between basic research and clinical experience to achieve any further results.

The round table that I had the honor to chair as a surgeon and as President of the European Burn Association at the European Tissue Repair Symposium is an example of this new approach to the problem. Of particular interest are the basic analogies which can be observed in the field of wound care in different ages and cultures. This is a typical example of how practical experience produces similar concepts and strategies under different conditions. In antique Greek or Egyptian care, an expert may have employed - even if concealed in magical belief - the same treatments that are used today such as hemostasis in the case of acute wound, detersion, antisepsis and coverage. This corresponds to our current practice and demonstrates that the main processes in wound healing remain the same regardless of whether hemostasis is obtained with hot ashes or fibrin glue, detersion is practiced with vinegar or H_2O_2, antisepsis is achieved with tea or sulfonamide, and a wound is covered with dry leaves or keratinocytes on a dermal-like layer produced with tissue engineering.

The expression "healing hand" makes us think of the fascinating volume by Guido Majino. His monogragh focuses in a modern way on the fundamental act of wound care in all the historical settings, stressing the main traditionals which are strikingly similar.

The objective of the monograph is to update our knowledge of enzymatic débridement obtained with collagenolitic enzymes which are so important in the context of the physiological mechanisms of wound repair and related to antibacterial action to abolish the substrates and to the chemotaxes of inflammatory cells. The protease/collagenase system is at the center of a complex series of phenomena involved in the healing of tegumental tissue wounds and in the modulation of the scarring process. We surgeons know very well that the quality of the final scar can determine therapeutic success. We therefore hope that continuing investigations by both basic scientists and surgeons will result in the much needed progress.

Professor Luigi Donati, Milan

Proteinases in Wound Repair

J. M. Davidson

Summary

The purpose of this brief discussion is to remind the reader that proteinases are not only involved in tissue remodeling, but that they have a broad range of roles in the process of tissue repair. Many of these enzymes are not stored, suggesting that their expression and activity can be modulated at the level of gene expression. Given the complexity and multiplicity of matrix metalloproteinases (MMP), much interest has developed toward understanding the activation pathways of these proteinases. Control of activation and inhibitor pathways offer additonal levels of manipulation. Although there has been some success in targeted deletions of metalloproteinase genes, these studies have not determined a precise biological role for the MMPs in wound repair. Crucial experiments will be necessary to determine when these molecules turn from friend to foe in the wound healing process.

Introduction

Proteolysis is an intrinsic component of tissue repair [6, 17]. From the inception of hemostasis, through débridement and control of infection, to the replacement of normal connective tissue architecture, a wide variety of enzymes come into play. During the last 10–15 years, our understanding of proteolysis and proteases has increased enormously. The metalloproteinase family has expanded from a single member, collagenase, to a family with perhaps more than a dozen members [1]. Likewise we have learned a great deal about the more traditional, serine proteinases and, perhaps more importantly, about the function of protease inhibitors at the mechanistic level. Proteases in wounds are initially delivered from the

Department of Pathology, Vanderbilt University School of Medicine and Research Service, Department of Veterans Affairs Medical Center, Nashville, Tennessee

Table 1. Are proteinases detrimental to wound repair?

Implications from wound fluids
  High proteolytic activity in wound fluid
    Elastase
    Gelatinase
  Fragmentation of macromolecules critical to cell attachment
  Inactivation of stimuli by chronic wound fluid

plasma or by blood-borne cells, but the tissue itself quickly begins to express many types of tissue-degrading or tissue-modifying activities.

In this paper and the articles that follow, the reader will come to appreciate the complexity of the control of proteolysis in the context of tissue repair. Not only is gene expression involved, but activation steps and the expression of proteinase inhibitors play an important role in determining the overall proteolytic activity profile of a particular wound at a particular stage. Proteinases in wounds can be friends or foes. Sufficient proteolysis must occur at the wound site to remove all necrotic material and dead infectious particles; however, excess or persistent proteolysis at the wound site will create a highly unfavorable environment for growth and migration of cells to repair the defect (Table 1). Hopefully, the next decade of basic and clinical research is going to put us in a position to manipulate these factors within the wound environment in order to obtain more satisfactory rates and quality of healing.

Hemostasis

From the initiating moment of tissue injury until well after the scar has matured, proteolytic activity plays a central role in the repair process (Table 2). The initial peptide bond cleavage events occur as elements of the coagulation cascade successively cleave zymogens into active forms to rapidly convert fibrinogen into fibrin and thereby reduce plasma and blood leakage. Excessive clot formation is counteracted by the actions of specific, circulating inhibitors such as antithrombin-III, and clot dissolution is catalyzed by the activation of plasmin via tissue- or urokinase-type plasminogen activators. In this way, proteinases set, within the first minutes after injury, the stage for the formation of the provisional matrix, a temporary scaffold at the wound site that will allow inflammatory and other blood-borne cells a migratory foothold. Coagulation and thrombosis are examples of incredibly tightly regulated

Table 2. Proteolytic events pervade the healing process

Key stages in wound repair

Hemostasis and thrombosis
  Coagulation cascade
  Fibrinolysis

Inflammatory cell activation
  Granulocyte
  Mast cell
  Macrophage

Tissue reconstruction
  Endothelium
  Epidermis/epithelium
  Fibroblast/myofibroblast

proteolytic events that have been well described as a distinct set of interrelated pathways.

Leukocytes and Their Proteinases (Table 3)

Hemostasis sets the stage for the activation of the next set of proteolytic events, the disinfection and débridement of the wound site by polymorphonuclear leukocytes. These cells, recruited by the activation of adhesive mechanisms on adjacent capillary endothelium, proceed to extravasate into the tissue space and the wound site under the influence of chemoattractants, at the same time releasing a tremendous barrage of granule-bound proteinases, particularly a group of serine proteinases and collagenase.

Table 3. Inflammatory cell proteinases

Granulocyte proteinases
  Serine proteinases
    Elastase
    Cathepsin G
    Proteinase 3
    Azurocidin
  Neutrophil collagenase (MMP-8)

Macrophage proteinases
  Collagenase (MMP-1)
  Metalloelastase (MMP-12)
  "Recycled" neutrophil elastase

Mast cell proteinases
  Tryptase (human)
  Chymase (mast cell protease I)
  Mast cell protease II (rat)

Mast Cells

Although a prominent participant in many inflammatory reactions, the repertoire of the mast cell is poorly understood. In their resting state these cells contain storage granules loaded with proteoglycan, histamine, and several serine proteinases. Upon activation, these granule contents are rapidly released, leading to massive increases in interstitial fluid and perfusion; however, the mast cell is not destroyed in the process of degranulation. Persistently activated mast cells, no longer distinctively marked by their metachromatic inclusions, can continue to mediate the inflammatory response and modulate cellular immune responses for days to weeks after degranulation. Chymase and tryptase are two serine proteinases present in mast cell granules. These enzymes have cleavage specificities similar to chymotrypsin and trypsin [9]. Carboxypeptidase A and B are present as well.

Neutrophils

Metalloproteinases. The matrix metalloproteinase MMP-8 (neutrophil collagenase) is a distinct gene product with higher catalytic efficiency for type III collagen [8]. Neutrophils may also express a newly described collagenase (collagenase-3; MMP-13) whose substrate specificity resembles that of the predominant isoform of rat collagenase.

Serine Proteinases. The neutrophil contains several enzymes of the serine proteinase class that attack peptide sequences in a host of proteins involved in wound repair, with the exception of triple helical collagen. The principal role of the neutrophil is defense and débridement; thus, these enzymes are crucial to the removal of peptides derived from killed, invading bacteria and spent host cells. Unlike most of the serine proteinases, the elastases are produced as active enzymes, being sequestered in secretory granules. A significant fraction of these enzymes is bound to the neutrophil surface, where it is protected from inhibition by proteinase inhibitors [10].

Elastase. The structure and mechanism of action of elastase is extremely well understood [15]. The primary sequence and substrate specificity of neutrophil elastase is very close to that of pancreatic elastase. Because it is one of the few enzymes that degrade intact, cross-linked elastin, elastase is undoubtedly involved in the destruction of elastic fibers, but it is equally capable of degrading core proteins of proteoglycans, growth factors, attachment factors, and a host of

4

other targets. In tissue space, elastase action is controlled by proteinase inhibitors, the best characterized of which is α1-antiproteinase (α1-antitrypsin; AAT) [11]. However, other proteinase inhibitors such as α2-macroglobulin must be active at sites of elastase action, since genetic deficiencies in AAT do not lead to wholesale destruction of tissue by inflammatory processes.

Neutrophil elastase is the major proteolytic activity released upon degranulation of polymorphonuclear leukocytes. It is probably the major enzyme involved in the débridement of damaged tissue. Imbalances in elastase activity have been shown to produce pathological changes in the lung (pulmonary emphysema) [2], and excess elastase activity appears to be associated with degradation of fibronectin and other molecules in the chronic wound [7].

Cathepsin G. Cathepsin G is another prominent constituent of the specific granule. It possesses a chymotrypsin-like substrate specificity and can also be classified as an elastase. Cathepsin G, like neutrophil elastase, has broad substrate specificity.

Proteinase 3 (PR-3). Proteinase 3, another distinct serine proteinase with connective tissue degrading activity, is also present in the specific granules of the neutrophil.

Azurocidin. Azurocidin, a molecule with close homology to the other neutrophil serine proteinases, has antibacterial activity but lacks catalytic activity [3].

Macrophages

Neutrophil Elastase. A serine-type elastase has been noted in macrophage populations, yet there has been no evidence that these cells can produce the enzyme. Interestingly, macrophages appear to have a specific uptake mechanism for released neutrophil elastase. The endocytosed elastase is apparently moved into a compartment wherein it may be recycled to the extracellular space.

Metalloelastase (MMP-12). MMP-12 is one of the newest members of the MMP family. The activity was first discovered in murine macrophages, and considerable effort was required to identify and isolate the homologous protein from human macrophages. This enzyme appears to represent the major elastolytic enzyme expressed by macrophages; however, like the serine elastolytic proteinases, the substrate specificity of

Table 4. "Tissue" proteinases

Epidermis
  Collagenase (MMP-1)
  Stromelysin-1,2 (MMP-3,10)
  Plasminogen activator (urokinase type)

Mesenchyme
  Collagenase (MMP-13)
  Stromelysin 1 (MMP-3)
  72-kDa gelatinase (MMP-2)
  92-kDa gelatinase (MMP-9)
  Plasminogen activator (uPA)

this enzyme is also quite broad, being able to attack many components of connective tissue, including proteins of the basement membrane.

Collagenase. Mature macrophages express the same collagenase gene product as fibroblasts (MMP-1). As with the fibroblast enzyme, proteolysis is principally directed at the interstitial collagens (I–III, V). Macrophages may also express the newly described collagenase-3 (MMP-13).

Fibroblast, Endothelial Proteinases

It is very clear that the cells of connective tissue can participate in remodeling through the expression of various proteinases. Most prominent are the expression of collagenase and plasminogen activators, but other classes of proteinases can have significant effects on matrix metabolism during development and repair (Table 4).

Proteinases As Activators

Digestion of peptide targets does not necessarily lead to their complete destruction. Proteolysis at the wound site will release a significant amount of biologically active material from higher molecular weight substrates. This includes chemotactically active fragments of matrix macromolecules, soluble forms of receptors that are cleaved from the cell surface, and cleavage of multifunctional chemokines (Table 5).

Procollagen C, N-Proteinases. There are two key enzymes involved in the conversion of soluble procollagen (types I, III, V, and XI) to tropocollagen by trimming off the C- and N-termini of the assembled procollagen molecules. Both of these enzymes are neutral metalloendopeptidases, and genetic defi-

Table 5. Proteinases as activators

Release of active peptides
  Chemotactic fragments of matrix components
  Soluble forms of receptors
  Cleavage of multifunctional chemokines
Processing of latent molecules
  Role of plasminogen activator in TGF-β activation
  Conversion of high molecular weight TGF-α/EGF precursors
  Procollagen conversion
   N-proteinase
   C-proteinase
    Conversion of types I–III procollagen
     Possible activity of c-peptide in cartilage
    Processing of lysyl oxidase
    Relationship to bone morphogenetic protein-1

TGF, transforming growth factor; EGF, epidermal growth factor.

ciency of the N-proteinase leads to a form of Ehlers-Danlos syndrome (type VII) with fragile skin. This is probably due to steric hindrance of normal collagen fibril assembly by the bulky, globular N-terminal domain. Subsequently, the disulfide linked C-termini of procollagen are processed by a c-proteinase. Cleavage is reportedly accelerated by the presence of an enhancer protein. The c-proteinase may be closely related to bone morphogenic protein-1 (BMP-1), which was previously known to be nonhomologous with the other, transforming growth factor-β (TGF-β) like BMPs. The primary structure of the c-proteinase identifies it as a member of the astacin family of metalloproteinases, which also includes tolloid protein. This is a proteinase gene first identified in *Drosophila,* and it is potentially involved in TGF-β activation.

Lysyl Oxidase Activation. Lysyl oxidase is not a proteinase, but an extracellular enzyme crucial to the cross-linking of collagen and elastin. This copper-dependent oxidase functions by deaminating e-amino groups on crucial lysyl residues in collagen and elastin, which, due to the protein's intrinsic assembly processes, condense to form very stable cross-link structures that are resistant to chemical and biological hydrolysis. Lysyl oxidase may be activated from its precursor form by an astacin-like proteinase.

Growth Factor Activation

Many cytokines are synthesized as latent precursors, thus activation represents another level of biological control.

Plasminogen Activator, Plasmin, Plasminogen Activator Inhibitor-1, and TGF-β. Plasminogen activator, a serine proteinase, exists in two forms: tissue type (tPA) and urokinase type (uPA), both of which are capable of cleaving plasminogen to its active form and thus setting off fibrinolysis. In addition, it has been shown that surface-associated uPA can be involved in a complex circuit, together with the mannose-6-phosphate receptor and plasmin, in the proteolytic activation of latent TGF-β to its active form. uPA is also associated with extracellular matrix degradation [12].

TGF-α Precursor. Both epidermal growth factor (EGF) and TGF-α are synthesized as large precursors with several similar growth factor domains. Cathepsin D, an aspartyl proteinase normally associated with lysosomes, can be found in the extracellular space, and it has the potential to act if the pH falls below about 6.5. Evidence has been presented to suggest that cathepsin D may play a role in processing of the EGF/TGF-α precursors. Kallikrein has also been mentioned as a processing enzyme for these proforms of growth factors [16].

Interleukin-1 Converting Enzyme and Programmed Cell Death. Programmed cell death (apoptosis) is certainly a normal aspect of wound healing. Cellularity rapidly rises and then falls at the wound site through this mechanism. It is clear that a number of proteins related to the interleukin-1 converting enzyme (ICE) are involved in the apoptotic pathway, and protease inhibitors, such as the crmA protein expressed by vaccinia virus, function by inhibiting the action of ICE-like enzymes and preventing death of the host cells. Interleukin-1 is synthesized as a precursor lacking a signal peptide for secretion. Intracellular processing leads to cytokine activation and may affect intracellular location.

Serine Proteinases

Plasminogen activator is certainly involved in proteolysis and fibrinolysis, but the tissue-type form of the enzyme is also associated with the cell surface and with surface activation events. tPA may also play a role in matrix degradation and the enhanced motility of cells. tPA expression is strongly induced by inflammatory mediators such as IL-1, while its expression is shut off by TGF-β. At the same time, TGF-β increases the expression of plasminogen activator inhibitor-1 (PAI-1), perhaps to increase the efficiency of proteolytic inhibition. Since tPA may be involved in TGF-β activation, this response would serve as a negative feedback loop controlling the activity of TGF-β [4].

Metalloproteinases

Collagenase. MMP-1 is the classic metalloproteinase that is absolutely required and specific for the degradation of triple helical types I, II, III, V, and XI collagens. Like other members of the MMP family, it contains a zinc atom at the active center and also requires calcium for full activity. Like other members of the MMP family, collagenase undergoes a complex activation, which may or may not require a proteolytic cleavage event [1]. Possible activating enzymes for collagenase include stromelysin-1 and plasminogen activator. The only known activity of collagenase is against the unique, triple helical substrate, and collagenase cleaves gelatin (denatured collagen) much less efficiently. Collagenase expression is under tight transcriptional regulation. Synthesis is strongly stimulated by agents that activate protein kinase C (e.g., phorbol esters, mitogenic growth factors, and TNF α/JL-1), and transcription is arrested by TGF-β. After tissue injury, collagenase is expressed in migrating keratinocytes, macrophages, and fibroblasts. A new human collagenase (MMP-13), probably corresponding to rat uterine collagenase, has recently been identified [5].

72-kDa Gelatinase(A): MMP-2. Unlike classic collagenase, other MMPs have much broader substrate specificity and expression patterns. This enzyme degrades denatured collagen and also attacks native collagens such as type IV, V, VII, X, as well as elastin and fibronectin. These properties have led to the proposal that MMP-2 is critically involved in cellular translocation through basement membrane structures as might occur in inflammation or tumor metastasis.

Stromelysin-1: MMP-3. Given this name because of broad substrate specificity, this enzyme is usually identified by a combination of its apparent molecular weight and caseinolytic activity. This enzyme was originally described as a cDNA clone from fibroblasts with a transformed phenotype, and its regulation is similar, but not identical, to collagenase. Stromelysin has been shown to be upregulated in migratory epidermis and mesenchymal cells scattered through granulation tissue. Stromelysin-1 activation may require the action of a surface-associated MMP (MT-MMP).

92-kDa Gelatinase(B): MMP-9. Unlike its 72-kDa counterpart, 92-kDa gelatinase tends to have a much more restricted pattern of expression and appears to be more tightly regulated at the level of gene expression. Activation of the zymogen form of the proteinase may require the previous activation by stromelysin-1.

Acid Proteinases

Cathepsin D. This enzyme is a lysosomal, aspartyl proteinase that is biochemically related to pepsin. Its pH optimum is in the range of 6.0–6.5. The enzyme may play a role beyond that of digestion of phagocytosed proteins, since this molecule, as many other lysosomal proteins, can find its way into the extracellular space where glycosylation directs uptake into lysosomes through the mannose-6-phosphate receptor. It is uncertain whether pericellular activity is part of a receptor-mediated recycling of enzyme plus substrate to the acidic environment of the lysosome, or whether there may be restricted compartments at the cell surface into which hydrogen ions are pumped to allow extracellular activity of this acid proteinase. In the past, cathepsin D activity has been associated with the processing of TGF-α and procollagen.

Cathepsin B, L. These lysosomal cysteine proteinases are significant from the perspective of intracellular degradation of macromolecules.

Epithelial Proteinases

These neutral metalloproteinases are largely associated with migratory events during the resurfacing of injury sites. With the exception of matrilysin, many of the same MMP genes activated in mesenchymal cells are called into play during epithelial migration in response to injury or remodeling [14]. The basic properties of the enzymes have already been mentioned, and the accompanying article by Parks, et al. (this volume) provides far greater detail on many aspects of these proteinases.

Collagenase. MMP-1 appears to be primarily expressed at the leading edge of the epidermal front.

Stromelysin 1. MMP-3 is co-expressed with collagenase, and perhaps a bit behind the leading edge.

Stromelysin 2. Stromelysin 2, an MMP closely related in structure and substrate specificity to MMP-3, is expressed more distal to the leading edge, at sites of basal lamina deposits and less hypertrophic epidermis. Expression, which probably differs because of variation in promoter structure, is possibly more associated with proliferative centers rather than migratory centers.

Matrilysin. Matrilysin, the smallest of the members of this class, is not known to be involved in wound healing processes. Expression of the enzyme is apparently confined to secretory epithelia (gut, endometrium) [13].

References

1. Birkedal-Hansen H (1995) Proteolytic remodeling of the extracellular matrix. Curr Opin Cell Biol 7 : 728–735
2. Davidson IM (1990) Biochemistry and turnover of lung interstitium. Eur Respir J 3 : 1048–1068
3. Elsbach P, Weiss J (1992) Oxygen-independent antimicrobial systems of phagocytes. In: Gallin JI, Goldstein IM, Snyderman R (eds) Inflammation: basic principles and clinical correlates. Raven, New York
4. Flaumenhaft R, Kojima S, Abe M et al (1993) Activation of latent transforming growth factor beta. Adv Pharmacol 24 : 51–76
5. Freije JM, Diez-Itza I, Balbin M et al (1994) Molecular cloning and expression of collagenase-3, a novel human matrix metalloproteinase produced by breast carcinomas. J Biol Chem 269 : 16766–16773
6. Gailit J, Clark RAF (1994) Wound repair in the context of the extracellular matrix. Curr Opin Cell Biol 6 : 717–725
7. Grinnell F, Zhu M (1994) Identification of neutrophil elastase as the proteinase in burn wound fluid responsible for degradation of fibronectin. J Invest Dermatol 103 : 155–161
8. Hasty KA, Pourmottabed T, Goldberg GI, et al (1990) Human neutrophil collagenase: a distinct gene product with homology to other matrix metalloproteinases. J Biol Chem 265 : 11421–11424
9. Katanuma N (1990) New biological functions of intracellular proteases and their endogenous inhibitors as bioreactants. Adv Enzyme Regul 30 : 377
10. Owen CA, Campbell MA, Sannes PL et al (1995) Cell surface-bound elastase and cathepsin G on human neutrophils: a novel, non-oxidative mechanism by which neutrophils focus and preserve catalytic activity of serine proteinases. J Cell Biol 131 : 775–789
11. Potempa J, Korzus E, Travis J (1994) The serpin superfamily of proteinase inhibitors: structure, function, and regulation. J Biol Chem 269 : 15957–15960
12. Rifkin DB (1992) Plasminogen activator expression and matrix degradation. Matrix [Suppl]1 : 20–22
13. Rogers WH, Osteen KG, Matrisian LM et al (1993) Expression and localization of matilysin, a matrix metalloproteinase, in human endometrium during the reproductive cycle. J Obstet Gynecol 168 : 253-260
14. Saarialho-Kere U, Pentland A, Birkedal-Hansen H et al (1994) Distinct populations of basal keratinocytes express stromelysin-1 and stromelysin-2 in chronic wounds. J Invest Dermatol 94 : 79–88
15. Travis J (1988) Structure, function, and control of neutrophil proteinases. Am J Med 84 : 37-42
16. Twining SS (1994) Regulation of proteolytic activity in tissues. Crit Rev Biochem Mol Biol 29 : 315 : 383
17. Westerhof W, Vanscheidt W (1994) Proteolytic enzymes and wound healing. Springer, Berlin Heidelberg New York

Interview

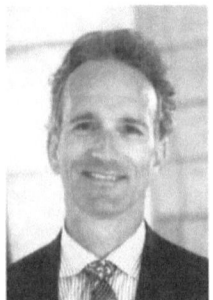

Chronic wounds – are they due more to a deficiency of certain growth factors and other cytokines or do they represent a state of overexpression of cytokines and proteases?

Davidson: Many chronic wounds appear to be locked in an inflammatory state. This suggests that there is excessive expression of inflammatory cytokines such as interleukin-1 and TNF-α that, as a consequence, elicit the elaboration of tissue-degrading enzymes. This excess of inflammatory proteinases could be destroying the growth factor signals necessary for wound maturation. Wounds of a diabetic and ischemic nature are probably not expressing sufficient levels of growth factors.

Is it reasonable to try and downregulate these proteinases?

Davidson: Absolutely. The key issue is to permit the physiological process of tissue remodeling while suppressing excess proteolysis. For example, if elastase and other serine proteinases are causing the pathological changes, then either low-molecular-weight inhibitors or the naturally occuring anti-proteinases could have a favorable effect. Selective MMP inhibitors or agents that block their expression might also be useful.

Which drugs are known to do so?

Davidson: The pharmaceutical industry has developed an enormous number of antielastases targeted at pulmonary disease, but they might also be effective in chronic wounds. α1-Antiproteinase was effective in one study. Tetracycline and its derivatives are fairly good MMP inhibitors. Several investigators have demonstrated the efficacy of peptide analogs in suppressing MMP-dependent proteolysis in the corneal ulcer, for example.

The Biochemical and Cellular Functions of the Matrix Metalloproteinases

G. Murphy

Summary

A number of metalloproteinases that degrade the extracellular matrix of connective tissues and three specific tissue inhibitors of metalloproteinases (TIMPs) have now been isolated, characterized, and cloned. Comparison of the enzyme sequences has allowed the delineation of domain structures, and initial studies have been carried out to assess the contribution of these domains to their biochemical and biologic properties, including activation, inhibition of TIMPs, and matrix binding. Such events represent the major levels of extracellular regulation of metalloproteinase activity, which is thought to be an important aspect of their control. Activation is probably a cell surface phenomenon, involving the plasminogen activator cascade or other membrane-associated mechanisms. The inhibitory action of TIMPs is postulated to be as important in activation as in the subsequent regulation of enzyme degradation of the matrix.

Regulation of the Matrix Metalloproteinases

The matrix metalloproteinases (MMPs) are a family of zinc-dependent enzymes that have the combined ability to degrade the macromolecules that constitute connective tissue matrices (Table 1). They are thought to be important in the cellular remodeling processes associated with both normal and pathological matrix turnover. Regulation of the MMPs occurs not only at the level of gene expression, but also extracellularly by cell surface-associated proteolytic cascades effecting activation, as well as by the action of highly specific inhibitors (tissue inhibitors of metalloproteinases: TIMPs).

Strangeways Research Laboratory, Worts' Causeway, Cambridge CBI 4RN, England

13

Table 1. Biochemical properties of human matrix metalloproteinases

Enzyme	MMP no.	Mol.wt. (proform)	Matrix proteins degraded
Collagenase	1	55 000	Single locus in native fibrillar collagens I, II, III; type-VIII, -X collagens
	8	75 000	Proteoglycan; gelatins (limited)
	13	65 000	Fibrillar collagen
Gelatinase A	2	72 000	Denatured collagens (gelatins); nonhelical regions fibrillar collagens
Gelatinase B (type-IV collagenase)	9	92 000	Specific locus type-IV collagens; type-V, -VII, -XI collagens; elastin
Stromelysin-1	3	57 000	Proteoglycan core protein; nonhelical regions type IV collagen (X-links); type-II, -IX collagens; fibronectin; laminin; gelatins (limited)
Stromelysin-2	10	57 000	Procollagens I, II, III; collagenase; gelatinase B
Matrilysin (pump)	7	28 000	Strong stromelysin-like activity; elastin
Stromelysin-3	11	51 000	Weak stromelysin-like activity
Metalloelastase	12	54 000	Similar to matrilysin; elastin
Membrane type	14	63 000	Progelatinase A

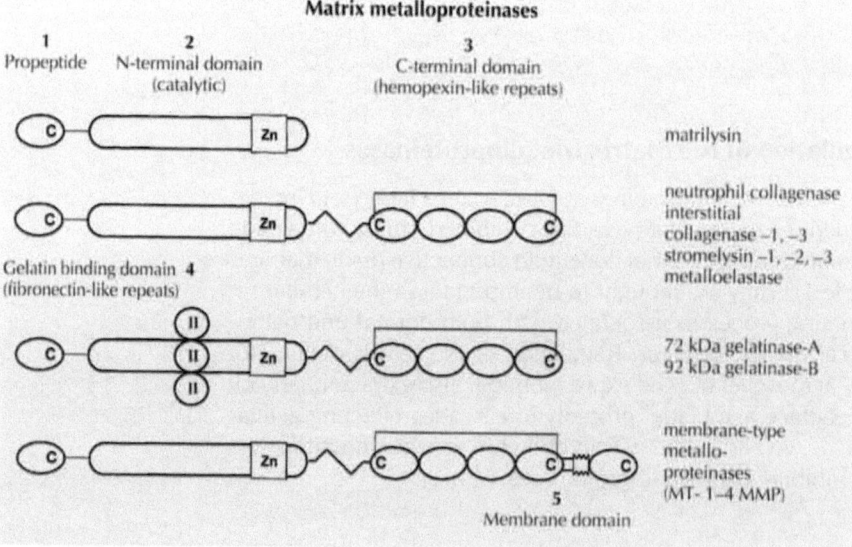

Fig. 1. Domain structures of the different classes of matrix metalloproteinases

Fig. 2. Role of domain structures in matrix metalloproteinase functions. GL-A, Gelatinase A

1. Propeptide (amino-terminal) — secretion process, latency

2. Catalytic domain (Zn, Ca binding) — self-cleavage, substrate cleavage, TIMP interaction

3. C-terminal domain — fibrillar collagen specificity (collagenase) collagen binding (collagenase/stromelysin) cell binding (gelatinase A) TIMP binding

4. Collagen binding domain (gelatinases A & B) — collagen binding kcat gelatinolysis type IV specificity

5. Membrane domain (MT-MMP) — cell association, GL-A/TIMP-2 binding

Matrix Metalloproteinase Structure

Our newly developed knowledge of the structure of the MMPs has led to the analysis of the role of definable domains in their biochemical and biological activity (Fig. 1) [1, 2]. The catalytic domain, which contains the active site Zn(II) and stabilizing Ca(II)-binding sites, is required for proteolytic activity and for the binding of the TIMPs. The latency of this domain is maintained in the proenzyme forms by the presence of a propeptide which is thought to donate a cysteine ligand to the active site Zn(II) (reviewed in [1]). All the MMPs except matrilysin have a C-terminal hemopexin/vitronectin-like domain which has a variety of roles, including collagen binding (collagenase and stromelysin), TIMP-1 binding (collagenase and gelatinases A and B), and membrane binding (gelatinase A). The gelatinases A and B have a further domain inserted into the catalytic domain, which shows close similarity to the type-II domain of fibronectin. Finally, the newly discovered membrane-type MMPs (MT MMPs) have a short spanning domain and a cytoplasmic tail C-terminal to the hemopexin domain (Fig. 2).

Matrix Metalloproteinase Activation

The precise mechanism by which the propeptide maintains latency is slowly being elucidated. The conserved sequence PRC GV/NPD is involved in interactions with the zinc of the adjoining catalytic domain. Other propeptide sequences apparently stabilize this interaction, since cleavage at sites N-terminal to the cysteine-containing motif will initiate autocatalytic activation. Sequential proteolysis of the propeptide is cer-

Fig. 3. Matrix metallo-proteinase activation. Sequential propeptide processing by exogenous proteinases often leads to self-cleavage

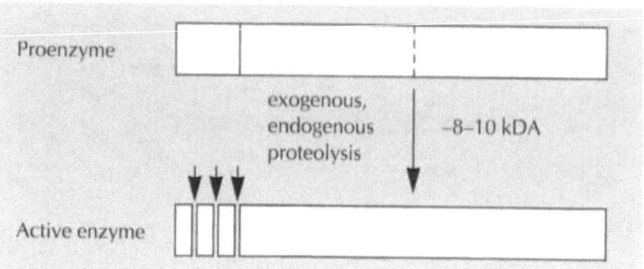

Proenzyme

exogenous, endogenous proteolysis

~8–10 kDA

Active enzyme

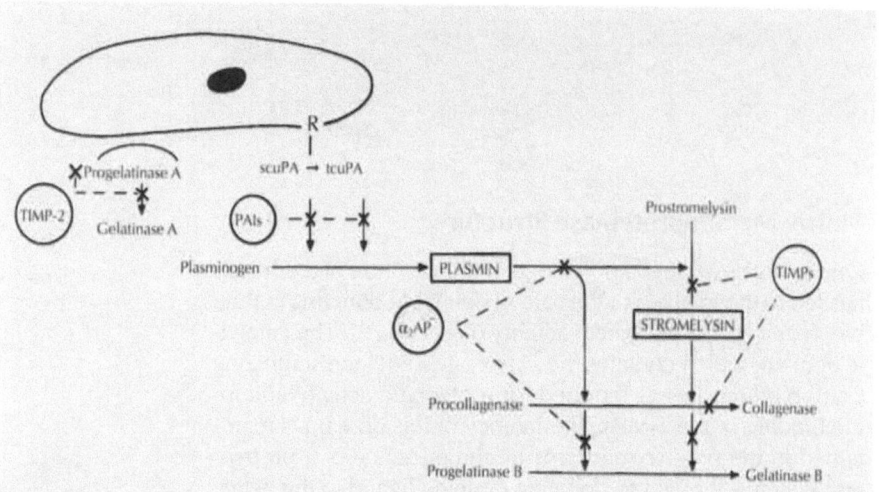

Fig. 4. Scheme for the pericellular proteolytic cascades responsible for matrix metalloproteinase activation. *PAI,* Plasminogen activator inhibitor; *UPA,* urokinase type plasminogen activator; *sc,* single chain; *tc,* two chain

tainly part of the activation process of MMPs and may involve proteinases of other classes or autolytic processing (Fig. 3). The activation of the collagenases, stromelysins-1 and -2, matrilysin, and gelatinase B may be initiated by plasmin, kallikreins, cathepsins B or G, or neutrophil-elastase. Plasmin has long been thought to be an important activator of these MMPs, and this concept has been supported by a number of studies using cell model systems. Plasmin generation and activity are known to occur largely at the cell surface, where both plasminogen and plasminogen activator are specifically bound (Fig. 4). It is likely that in localized pericellular regions the action of α2 anti-plasmin is limited, allowing plasmin activity. Stromelysins-1 and -2, which can be sequestered on the collagenous matrix, may be activated by plasmin and can then effect activation of collagenases and gelatinase B. TIMPs may regulate the activation process, since it has been shown that they can slow down or prevent the autocatalytic cleavages that occur.

Unlike the other MMPs, gelatinase A is not efficiently activated by either plasmin or trypsin. This enzyme can be activated

Fig. 5. Tissue inhibitors of metalloproteinases

TIMP-1	TIMP-2	TIMP-3
29 kDA glycoprotein	22 kDA non-glycosylated	24 kDA glycoprotein/ nonglycosylated
binds to progelatinase B	binds to progelatinase A	deposited in ECM

Produced by many connective tissue cells, occurs in body fluids, tissue extracts

Inhibit ACTIVE matrix metalloproteinases with 1:1 stoichiometry

Tight, non-covalent binding

No activity upon other metalloendopeptidases

6 loop disulphide bonded structure. About 40% sequence similarity

N-terminal 3 loops essential for activity

Fig. 6. Summary of TIMP-matrix metalloproteinase domain interactions

1. The N-terminal domain of TIMPs binds and inhibits active matrix metalloproteinases.
2. They no longer bind to progelatinases
3. Differences in the rate of binding of TIMPs with different MMPs is determined by *different* binding sites on the MMPs' N- and C-terminal domains for sites on the TIMPs' C-terminal domains.

by association with the cell membrane of many cell types and specific cleavage by MT MMPs (Fig. 4). Studies to date suggest that TIMP-2 is a very important regulator of this activation process, whereas TIMP-1 is not effective.

Inhibition of Matrix Metalloproteinases

The TIMPs are the major physiological inhibitors of the MMPs [3]. Three members of this family have been isolated and shown to have closely related structures and properties (Fig. 5). The TIMPs form tight binding complexes with the active MMPs with K_ds in the 10^{-9}–10^{-12} M range. They have 12 identically conserved cysteine residues forming six disulfide bonds which confer marked stability to the molecules. A two-domain structure of three loops each can be delineated, and it has been shown that the N-terminal three loops can fold independently and function as an efficient inhibitor of most MMPs. The C-terminal loops are involved in initial interactions with the enzyme (Fig. 6). Mutagenesis studies have indicated that the inhibitors present an extended contact surface to the MMPs, as has been shown for the serine proteinase inhibitors, the serpins. Catalytic activity of the MMP is not itself required for TIMP binding, merely access to the active site cleft.

Conclusions

The importance of the MMPs, both in the large-scale determination of tissue structure and in the relationships between connective tissue cells and their matrix, is now clear. Future work will determine precisely how they are involved in the key role of the extracellular matrix in determining cell behavior. An understanding of the regulatory mechanisms for MMP activity is consequently a central aspect of the elucidation of their importance in both physiological and pathological processes.

References

1. Birkedal-Hansen H (1995) Curr Opin Cell Biol 7 : 728–735
2. Docherty AJP, O'Connell J, Crabbe T, Angal S, Murphy G (1992). Trends Biotechnol 10 : 200–207
3. Murphy G, Willenbrock F (1995). Methods Enzymol 248 : 496–509

Interview

The balance of metalloproteinases and their inhibitors plays an important role. Is there any evidence that this balance is disturbed in impaired wound healing?

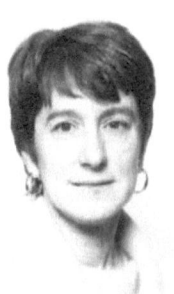

Murphy: Recent data has shown that fibrotic diseases are associated with an over expression of TIMP-1.

Is there anything known about systemic drugs which enhance or inhibit metalloproteinase activity?

Murphy: Some clinical studies have used tetracyclines, which act in part as metalloproteinase inhibitors, in the treatment of periodontal disease. Tetracycline derived inhibitors reduce enzyme activity and prevent radiographic destruction in a rat model of arthritis.

Is anything known about the influence of topical drugs on the MMP-TIMP balance?

Murphy: In model systems, e.g., corneal ulceration, chick chorioallantoic membrane or rat corneal angiogenesis, topical use of low molecular weight inhibitors of matrix metalloproteinases do seem to be effective.

Further Reading

Greenwald RA, Golub LM (eds) (1994) Inhibition of matrix metalloproteinases – therapeutic potential. Ann NY Acad Sci 732

Interstitial Collagenase in the Healing Epidermis

W. C. Parks

Summary

An invariable feature of wounded skin, whether the lesion is healing normally or chronic, is the expression of interstitial collagenase by migrating basal keratinocytes. Collagenase is a member of the matrix metalloproteinase family of enzymes and is the principal human enzyme which cleaves native fibrillar collagen. This proteinase may serve to accelerate the movement of keratinocytes during repair; however, its overexpression at the migrating front of the epidermis may actually impair healing in chronic ulcers. This potential inhibitory effect of human collagenase in nonhealing lesions is both spatially removed and mechanistically distinct from débridement of necrotic tissues overlying the wound bed by the topical application of bacterial collagenase and other broad-acting proteinases.

Introduction

Wound healing is an orderly process which involves inflammation, re-epithelialization, matrix deposition, and tissue remodeling. In most injuries, especially chronic wounds, healing is accompanied by inflammation, angiogenesis, and the formation of granulation tissue. Because degradation of extracellular matrices is needed to remove damaged tissue and provisional matrices and to permit vessel formation and cell migration, these normal remodeling processes require the activity of various proteinases. In chronic or nonhealing wounds, however, overexpression of proteinases likely contributes to the underlying pathology and may actually inhibit normal repair processes. Various cell types contribute numerous, distinct proteases that affect tissue restructuring during healing, and matrix metalloproteinases (MMPs), in particular interstitial collagenase, seemingly play a critical role in various stages of cutaneous repair.

Division of Dermatology, Jewish Hospital, Washington University School of Medicine, 216 S. Kingshighway, St. Louis, MO 63110 USA

Metalloproteinases

Metalloproteinases constitute a family of matrix-degrading enzymes with the combined capacity to degrade nearly all components of the extracellular matrix and are categorized by their capacity to degrade various extracellular matrix substrates, properties which are conferred by unique domains within the structure of the enzymes [1–3]. Members include three collagenases, two stromelysins, two gelatinases, matrilysin, metalloelastase, and a membrane-type MMP which may be involved in pro-enzyme activation [4]. Similar to other types of proteinases, MMPs are activated after secretion, and their enzymatic activity can be regulated by soluble inhibitors, such as the tissue inhibitors of metalloproteinases (TIMP-1, -2, and -3). To date, 11 different MMPs representing 11 distinct gene products have been characterized, and it is likely that additional members of this gene family will be identified in the future.

Interstitial collagenase[1] (also called collagenase-1 or MMP-1), the best-characterized, and historically oldest MMP, catalyzes the initial step in the degradation of fibrillar type-I and -III collagens, which together comprise the most abundant components of the dermal extracellular matrix. (To date, the other human collagenases, MMP-8 and MMP-13, have not been shown to be as widely produced as interstitial collagenase). The fibrillar collagens, which also include cartilage type-II collagen, are large, insoluble, protease-resistant matrix molecules that provide strength to tissues such as skin, tendons, and bone. Because collagenases are the only known mammalian proteinases that can cleave fibrillar collagens in their triple helical domains, and because the collagens are so abundant in many tissues, including the skin, the activity of these MMPs is essential for effective interstitial matrix remodeling. Collagenases do not degrade native type-I collagen but rather cleave the molecule at a single site located about three fourths of the distance from the N-terminus of the collagen molecule. At physiologic temperature (37° C), the two fragments of collagenase digestion denature spontaneously into gelatin peptides, which can be completely degraded by a variety of enzymes.

MMPs are involved in numerous normal and disease processes, but these enzymes also participate in unwanted events,

---

[1] Please note that human interstitial collagenase (referred to as collagenase in this chapter) is an enzyme distinct from bacterial collagenase. This latter enzyme, which is used in certain débridement ointments, has a very broad substrate specificity and can completely degrade fibrillar collagens.

such as tumor growth, arthritis, and essentially any condition associated with chronic inflammation. Because MMPs likely play a critical role in wound repair, we began to study the pattern of enzyme expression in human wounds of various etiologies. Our findings revealed that the basal epidermis is a prominent source of collagenase. We believe that interstitial collagenase serves an essential role in normal repair, but that its overexpression in chronic ulcers may actually hinder healing.

Methods

Tissue Specimens

Over 100 formalin-fixed, paraffin-embedded histological specimens were obtained from the Department of Pathology, Washington University School of Medicine. These samples included ulcerated pyogenic granuloma and nonhealing ulcers of various etiologies, such as stasis, decubitus, and nonspecific ulcers, and pyoderma gangrenosum. Nonspecific ulcers were characterized by overt inflammation and granulation tissue. To study metalloproteinase expression in acute wounds, we obtained specimens from Dr. John Olerud at the University of Washington School of Medicine [5, 6].

In Situ Hybridization

To assess the location and cell source of metalloproteinase production in human wounds, we used in situ hybridization as described in detail by Prosser et al. [7]. Basically, in situ hybridization is a modified histochemical assay which allows for the detection of specific mRNAs within a tissue section. Thus, this procedure allows for the direct determination of which cell type in a heterogeneous tissue is actively expressing a specific gene product. The method relies on the autoradiographic visualization of hybridized complexes of cellular mRNA with a radioactive nucleic acid probe.

Tissue sections were cut at 5 μm, deparaffinized, and rehydrated. All sections were treated briefly with nuclease-free proteinase K to loosen the constraints of intracellular cross-links caused by fixation, thereby enhancing diffusibility of probes to their target mRNAs. All sections were washed in a freshly prepared triethanolamine buffer containing acetic anhydride to reduce potential nonspecific binding sites. Sections were then covered with a sufficient volume of hybridization buffer containing ^{35}S-labeled probe, and the slides were incubated overnight to allow sufficient time for the probe to find and react with its target. After hybridization, the slides were washed extensively to remove the unhybridized probe. The probes are long stretches of nucleic acid molecules that are synthesized in the lab and whose sequences are specific for the various metalloproteinases.

Washed slides were dipped in a thick layer of photographic emulsion and stored for 5–21 days. During this period, the radioactive probe decayed, and the β particles interacted with and activated the silver grains in the emulsion. These activated grains were developed by conventional photographic processing and, when illuminated by dark-field microscopy, were seen as bright white dots. The slides were counterstained with hematoxylin and eosin to reveal tissue morphology.

Immunohistochemistry

To verify that cells expressing metalloproteinase mRNA also produced the protein and to map the location of cell populations, sections serial to those used for in situ hybridization were immunostained for various metalloproteinases or components of the basement membrane (type-IV collagen or laminin) by the peroxidase-antiperoxidase technique. Highly purified, specific antibodies were used for all assays. Controls were performed with the appropriate preimmune serum.

Keratinocyte Culture

Human keratinocytes were obtained from reduction mammoplasties or abdominoplasties. The subcutaneous fat and deep dermis were removed, the skin was cut into thin pieces, and the tissue was incubated overnight in trypsin as described by Pentland et al. [8]. The next morning, the epidermis was separated from the dermis, and the basal keratinocytes were scraped into growth medium. Under these conditions, the keratinocytes actually differentiate and stratify similarly to intact skin. Cells were grown on various concentrations of either purified type-I collagen or Matrigel (Collaborative Research, Inc., Bedford, Mass.), which is a mixture of basement membrane proteins. After 72 h, the medium was collected, and the levels of accumulated interstitial collagenase were measured by an enzyme-linked immunosorbant assay (ELISA) [6]. This assay has nanogram sensitivity, is specific for collagenase, and measures total enzyme present, whether free or bound to TIMP or substrate, and whether in an inactive or an active form.

Results

Interstitial Collagenase Is Produced by Basal Keratinocytes in Wounded Skin

Many studies have shown that collagenase is present in the wound environment [9, 10], and it has often been assumed that the enzyme is produced primarily by fibroblasts, macrophages, and other cells within the granulation tissue [11]. Indeed, collagenase is expressed in fibroblasts and macrophages in human burns [12] and in some samples of wounded skin and necrobiotic disorders [6, 12–14]. However, using in situ hybridization and immunohistochemistry assays, we found that collagenase was expressed in the dermis in fewer than 50% of the more than 100 samples we examined representing various forms of chronic wounds, including decubitus, sepsis, nonspecific ulcers and pyogenic granuloma, and when detected in dermal cells, the expression was typically low and confined to just a few cells [6, 13]. Furthermore, collagenase was not produced in dermal cells in samples of acute human wounds or in healthy skin.

In contrast, basal keratinocytes as the migrating front of re-epithelialization are the predominant source of collagenase during active wound repair (Fig. 1). Furthermore, we have found that collagenase expression by migrating keratinocytes is an invariable feature of a disrupted epidermis, both as a consequence of normal wound healing by secondary intention and in ulceration resulting from a variety of disease processes. This enzyme is also expressed by migrating basal keratinocytes in full-thickness burn wounds [12]. Although collagenase is always produced by epidermal cells at the wound edge, the level of expression varies considerably among wound types. In chronic ulcers, we typically saw very high levels of expression in the basal keratinocytes, and in these samples we often saw expression in the underlying dermis (Fig. 1C). In pyogenic granulomas, which are small benign ulcers that can heal spontaneously, we saw strong expression of collagenase mRNA, which was strictly confined to the migrating basal keratinocytes and noticeably weaker than that seen in many chronic specimens (Figs. 1A, B and 2). In acute wounds, the signal for collagenase mRNA was still limited to the basal epidermis but was much weaker than that seen in any other sample [6]. Collectively, these observations indicate that levels of collagenase produced in the epidermis are much greater in nonhealing wounds than in normally healing wounds and suggest that overexpression of this MMP may impair healing (see Fig. 7).

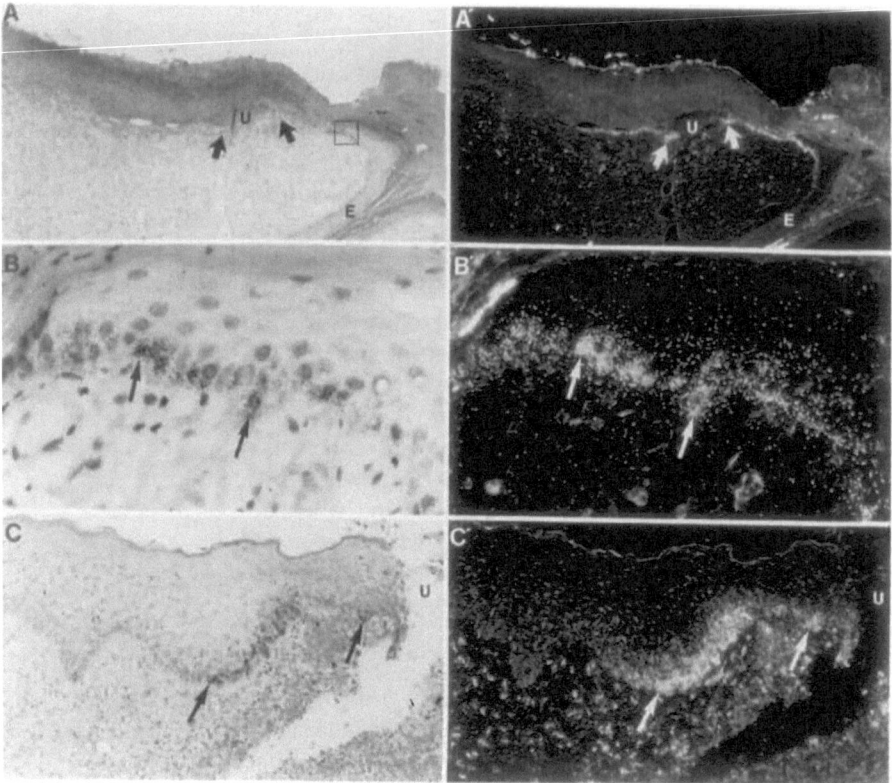

Fig. 1 A–C. Collagenase is expressed by basal keratinocytes at the leading edge of re-epithelialization in ulcers. **A** and **A′** Paired bright- and dark-field views of a sample of pyogenic granuloma hybridized with an ^{35}S-labeled antisense RNA probe specific for collagenase mRNA. An ulcerated area (U) is indicated, and collagenase-positive keratinocytes are seen on both sides of the ulcer (arrows). The intensity of the signal for collagenase mRNA diminishes with increasing distance from the ulcer. **B** and **B′** High-magnification views of the area indicated by the box in A. Prominent collagenase expression is localized only to basal keratinocytes (arrows). **C** and **C′** Bright- and dark-field views of a section of a nonspecific ulcer hybridized for collagenase mRNA. Note the intense collagenase expression by basal keratinocytes (arrows) forming the leading edge of re-epithelialization adjacent to the ulcer. In this specimen, collagenase is also expressed by underlying dermal fibroblasts. No signal was detected on any sample hybridized with a sense RNA probe (not shown)

The degradative activity of collagenase in the dermis and epidermis may be involved in distinct healing processes. Keratinocytes may degrade dermal collagen to aid migration and promote re-epithelialization, whereas stromal collagenase activity may effect tissue remodeling associated with granulation and scar formation. Since epidermal repair is common to all wounds and is ongoing when healing is most apparent, it is reasonable that collagenase was expressed by migrating kerati-

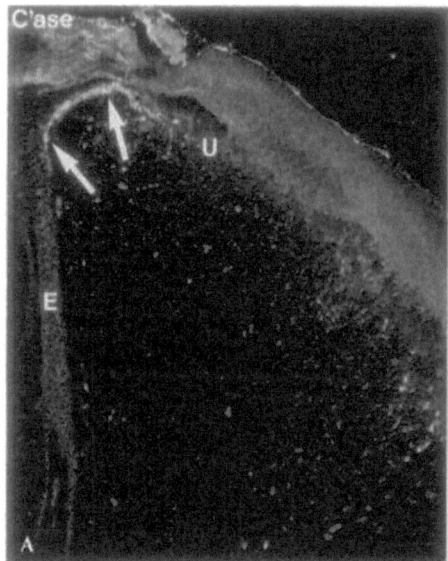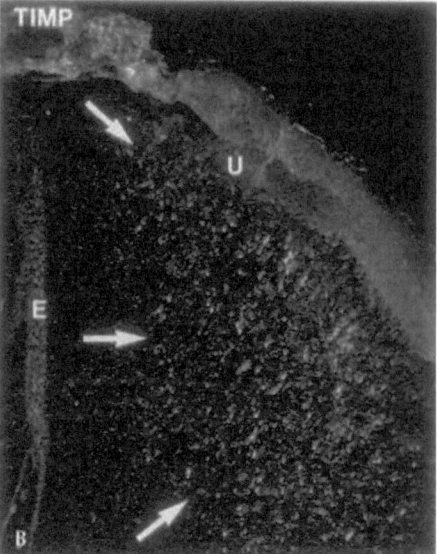

nocytes in all samples we examined. In contrast, the mass of granulation and scar tissue varies among wounds, and the resolution of these transient tissues occurs during defined periods of repair. Thus, although collagenase may be needed to remodel the dermal matrix, it may not be expressed, and hence detected, at all stages of repair.

Collagenase and TIMP-1 in Wound Healing

Collagenolytic activity is regulated, in part, by natural inhibitors, particularly the tissue inhibitor of metalloproteinases-1, or TIMP-1. Although cell-culture studies have shown that keratinocytes are capable of secreting TIMP-1 [15] and that most collagenase-producing cells also make TIMP-1, we have found that TIMP-1 mRNA does not colocalize with collagenase mRNA in migrating keratinocytes in chronic wounds (Fig. 2) [13]. Typically, TIMP-1 is expressed by stromal or perivascular cells, usually away from sites of collagenase expression. This distinct localization of enzyme and inhibitor suggests that keratinocyte-derived collagenase acts without impedance from TIMP-1, and this actually makes sense.

As for most biological processes, matrix degradation is a precise event. Proteases are produced and released on demand from cells which are activated to degrade matrix proteins. By means of specific cell-surface receptors, the cell recognizes a particular matrix molecule and is instructed to produce the

Fig. 2 A, B. Collagenase and TIMP-1 are expressed in distinct sites. Shown are serial sections hybridized for collagenase (C´ase) or TIMP-1m RNAs.
A Collagenase-positive basal keratinocytes are detected only at the migrating front of epithelium *(arrows).*
B In contrast, TIMP-positive cells are found within the underlying granulation tissue (bordered by arrows), but not in epidermis *(E).*
U, ulcerated area

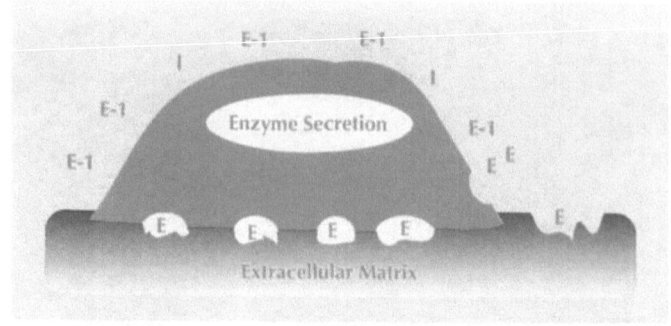

Fig. 3. Pericellular degradation of extracellular matrix. By means of precise interactions, cells recognize and adhere to specific extracellular matrix molecules. If the cell is activated for tissue remodeling, the appropriate proteolytic enzyme (E) is released into pericellular compartments where degradation would occur. Excess and "used" enzymes would be released into the tissue space and rapidly neutralized by specific inhibitor proteins (I)

appropriate metalloproteinase. The protease is released in a protected pericellular compartment, where it degrades its substrate (Fig. 3). Thus, TIMPs are present in the tissue environment to neutralize "used" proteinases, thereby preventing excessive and unwanted degradation away from the sites of metalloproteinase production (Fig. 3).

Alterations in the Tissue Environment Induce Collagenase Production by Basal Keratinocytes

The interaction of keratinocytes with the dermal matrix, in particular type-I collagen, may provide an early and critical signal to initiate the epithelial response to wounding. An interesting aspect of the epithelial expression of interstitial collagenase in wounded skin is that the enzyme is not produced in nonulcerated samples [6, 13, 16]. Also, our in situ hybridization studies clearly show that only basal keratinocytes, and not the more differentiated cells of the stratum spinosum and stratum granulosum, express collagenase mRNA (see Fig. 1B). The confinement of collagenase expression to the basal epidermal cells suggests that disruption of the basement membrane and subsequent exposure of keratinocytes to the underlying dermal stroma is apparently a critical determinant for the induction of epidermal collagenolytic activity.

Basal keratinocytes normally rest on a basement membrane composed of laminin, entactin, proteoglycans, type-IV collagen, and other matrix proteins [17]. In response to wounding, keratinocytes migrate from the edge of the wound under a provisional matrix of fibrin and fibronectin [18] and over the dermis, which includes structural macromolecules, such as type-I collagen, microfibrils, and elastin, distinct from those in the basement membrane. Loss of contact with the basement membrane and establishment of new cell-matrix interactions with components of the dermal and provisional matrices may

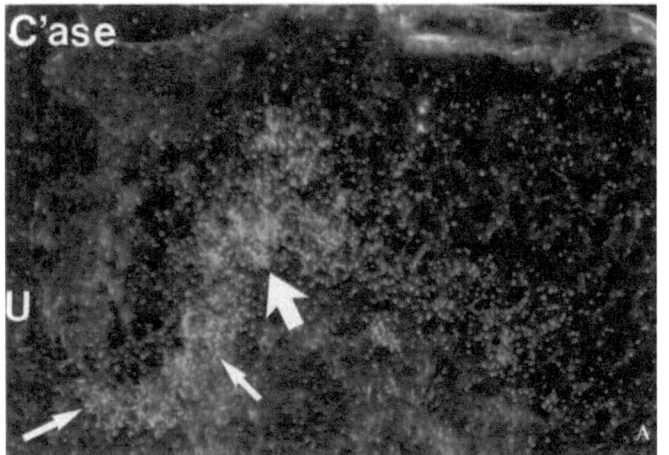

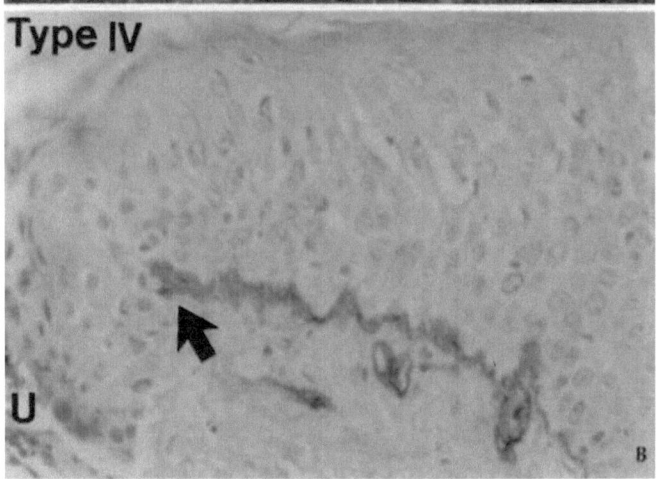

Fig. 4 A, B. Keratinocytes expressing collagenase are not in contact with basement membrane. Serial sections from a specimen of a nonspecific chronic ulcer *(U)* were (**A**) hybridized for collagenase (C´ase) or were (**B**) immunostained for type-IV collagen. The extent of basal lamina is marked by large arrows. Most collagenase-positive keratinocytes *(small arrows)* are not in contact with basement membrane, but rather are migrating over the dermal matrix. Signal for collagenase mRNA diminishes rapidly in areas with intact basal lamina

be a critical determinant that alters keratinocyte phenotype and induces collagenase production. Indeed, our in vivo observations show that collagenase-positive keratinocytes are not in contact with an intact basement membrane, as demonstrated by immunostaining for type-IV collagen and laminin-1, and migrate over the dermal wound matrix (Fig. 4).

Reflecting this in vivo relationship between metalloproteinase expression and contact with the dermis, collagenase production is induced in human basal keratinocytes grown on a surface coated with native type-I collagen (Fig. 5), the most abundant component of dermal matrix. In contrast, components of the basement membrane (Fig. 5) and other proteins of the interstitial matrix do not affect collagenase expression. Furthermore, the inductive effect of collagen is dependent on its native fibrillar structure. Although keratinocytes will adhere to

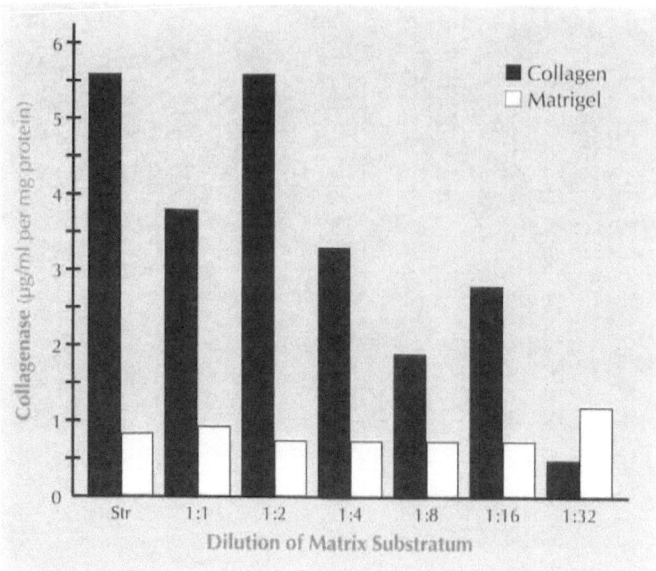

Fig. 5. Expression of interstitial collagenase is induced in human keratinocytes grown on native type-I collagen. Normal human keratinocytes were isolated and cultured on dishes coated with either fibrillar type-I collagen or basement membrane proteins (Matrigel). Collagen was added at 750 µg/ml (Str, straight) and diluted serially to 12 µg/ml. Matrigel was added in concentrations ranging from 3000 µg/ml (Str) to 47 µg/ml. After the cells reached confluence, the medium was changed and collected 72 h later. The levels of accumulated interstitial collagenase were measured by a competitive ELISA

denatured collagen (gelatin), collagenase production is turned on in response to this substrate [19]. In other studies, keratinocytes were shown to recognize and migrate on type-I collagen substratum, and this interaction results in enhanced collagenase production [20]. Collectively, these studies demonstrate a key role for type-I collagen in initiating keratinocyte collagenase synthesis in the epithelial response to wounding.

In addition to encountering different extracellular matrix proteins, migrating keratinocytes also express a distinct pattern of matrix-binding receptors, and these may also be involved in regulation of collagenase production. These receptors, called integrins, are heterodimeric surface molecules composed of distinct α and β chains that cells use to attach to various matrix proteins or to each other. Integrins are also used by cells to move or to migrate over the extracellular matrix. Various groups have shown that the collagen-binding integrin, $\alpha2\beta1$, is expressed on basal keratinocytes in intact skin and in epidermal cells at the wound edge [21–24]. In addition, keratinocytes at the wound edge selectively express other integrins, such as $\alpha5\beta1$, which are characteristic of migrating cells and which can bind proteins that are abundant in the wound bed. Since basal epidermal cells are not normally in contact with type-I collagen, it is tempting to speculate that the basal production of the collagen-binding integrin $\alpha2\beta1$ keeps keratinocytes primed and ready to respond to injury and induces the expression of collagenase. On the other hand, newly expressed integrins at the migrating front may be used by cells for migration.

Role of Collagenase in Wound Repair

The invariant and prominent production of interstitial collagenase by basal keratinocytes in both acute and chronic wounds indicates that this metalloproteinase serves a critical and required role in re-epithelialization, rather than in dermal remodeling. As stated, collagenase cleaves fibrillar collagen, which denatures at body temperature to gelatin. Since the $\alpha2\beta1$ integrin receptor for type-I collagen binds native collagen much more tightly than it does gelatin [25], interstitial collagenase may aid in dissociating keratinocytes from the collagen-rich matrix and thereby promote efficient locomotion over the dermal and provisional matrices. Thus, in the cutaneous wound-healing response, collagenase may serve a beneficial function, unlike its potentially destructive role in arthritis and vascular disease [26, 27].

In addition to interstitial collagenase, we found that two other MMPs, stromelysin-1 and stromelysin-2, which are distinct gene products yet degrade the same matrix components, are produced by separate populations of basal keratinocytes (Fig. 6) [28]. Significantly, and unlike the invariable expression of

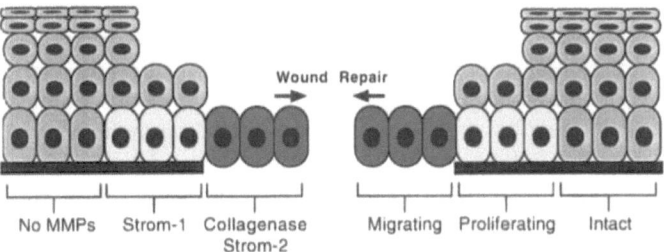

Fig. 6. Distinct spatial pattern of metalloproteinase expression in wounded epidermis. Three populations of keratinocytes are recognized in the healing epidermis: (a) the migrating front of basal keratinocytes which are not in contact with the basement membrane, (b) a hyperproliferative region of basal cells which are in contact with the basement membrane and which produces the nonproliferating migrating cells, and (c) intact skin at some variable distance from the wound area. Collagenase is prominently and invariably expressed by migrating basal keratinocytes in all wounds, whether acute or chronic, characterized by disruption of the basement membrane. Stromelysin-1 and -2 (Strom-1, Strom-2) are also expressed in the epidermis, but by a functionally distinct subpopulation of basal keratinocytes. In addition, the stromelysins are not expressed in all wounds, and thus their proteolytic activity may actually be a detriment to proper wound healing in chronic ulcers. No metalloproteinases (MMPs) are expressed in intact epidermis

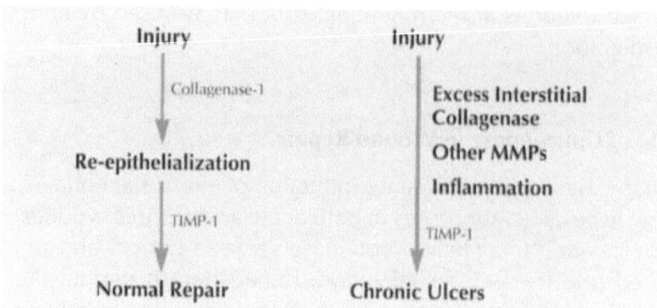

Fig. 7. Balance of metalloproteinases and inhibitors in normal and chronic wounds. Collagenase is expressed by migrating keratinocytes in all wounds, whether acute or chronic. The proper, regulated levels of collagenase may promote re-epithelialization by assisting in migration. Antiproteinases, such as TIMP-1, present in the wound fluid, would neutralize collagenase after remodeling, thereby preventing excess degradation. In chronic ulcers, however, noticeably more collagenase is expressed by basal keratinocytes, and additional proteinases, namely stromelysin-1 and stromelysin-2, are also produced. This localized overproduction of metalloproteinases, along with continued inflammation and underproduction of TIMPs, may lead to excess matrix degradation and impaired healing

collagenase, the stromelysins were detected only in chronic wounds. Thus, the production of these MMPs may represent unregulated proteinase production that actually contributes to the inability of certain ulcers to heal. Appropriate and efficient re-epithelialization may require the proper balance of proteinases and inhibitors (Fig. 7). In a chronic wound, however, overexpression of collagenase, coupled with the additional production of stromelysins and the underproduction of TIMPs [29], may impair healing by destroying newly deposited matrix and cytokines and by disrupting cell-cell interactions. Further studies will be needed to accurately determine the role of the various metalloproteinases that are expressed in temporal and site-specific patterns during wound repair.

Acknowledgements. I would like to thank Dr. Howard G. Welgus, who has collaborated with me on all our wound-healing studies; Dr. Ulpu Saarialho-Kere, currently at the University of Helsinki, who, as a postdoctoral fellow in my lab, made essentially all of our in vivo findings on metalloproteinase expression in wounds; Dr. Alice Pentland, who has been instrumental in helping us establish keratinocyte cultures; and our past and current fellows, Drs. Barry D. Sudbeck, Sarah Dunsmore, Brian Pilcher, and Steven O. Kovacs, for their contributions on the role and regulation of collagenase expression in basal keratinocytes. Our wound-healing research has been supported by grants HL-48762, HL-29594, and AM35805 from the National Institutes of Health, by a grant from Monsanto-Searle, Inc., and by the generous support of the Dermatology Foundation.

References

1. Parks WC, Sires UI (1995) Matrix metalloproteinases and skin biology. Curr Opin Dermatol 3 : 240–247
2. Woessner JF (1991) Matrix metalloproteinases and their inhibitors in connective tissue remodeling. FASEB J 5 : 2145–2154
3. Birkedal-Hansen H, Moore WGI, Bodden MK, Windsor LJ, Birkedal-Hansen B, DeCarlo A, Engler JA (1993) Matrix metalloproteinases: a review. Crit Rev Oral Biol Med 4 : 197–250
4. Sato H, Takino T, Okada Y, Cao J, Shinagawa A, Yamamoto E, Seiki M (1994) A matrix metalloproteinase expressed on the cell surface of invasive tumour cells. Nature 370 : 61–65
5. Olerud JE, Gown AM, Bickembach J, Dale B, Odland GF (1988) An assessment of human epidermal repair in elderly normal subjects using immunohistochemical methods. J Invest Dermatol 90 : 845–850
6. Saarialho-Kere UK, Kovacs SO, Pentland AP, Olerud J, Welgus HG, Parks WC (1993) Cell-matrix interactions modulate interstitial collagenase expression by human keratinocytes actively involved in wound healing. J Clin Invest 92 : 2858–2866
7. Prosser IW, Stenmark KR, Suthar M, Crouch EC, Mecham RP, Parks WC (1989) Regional heterogeneity of elastin and collagen gene expression in intralobar arteries in response to hypoxic pulmonary hypertension as demonstrated by in situ hybridization. Am J Pathol 135 : 1073–1088
8. Pentland AP, Jacobs Sc, Mahoney M, Holzman MJ (1990) Ultraviolet light potentiates histamine-induced release of prostaglandin in cultured human keratinocytes: a mechanism for irradiation erythema. J Clin Invest 86 : 566–574
9. Ågren MS, Taplin CJ, Woessner JF, Eaglstein WH, Mertz PM (1992) Collagenase in wound healing: effect of wound age and type. J Invest Dermatol 99 : 709–714
10. Buckley-Sturrock A, Woodward SC, Senior RM, Griffin GL, Klagsbrun M, Davidson JM (1989) Differential stimulation of collagenase and chemotactic activity in fibroblasts derived from rat wound repair tissue and human skin by growth factors. J Cell Physiol 138 : 70–78
11. Porras-Reyez BH, Blair HC, Jeffrey JJ, Mustoe TA (1991) Collagenase production at the border of granulation tissue in a healing wound: macrophage and mesenchymal collagenase production in vivo. Connect Tissue Res 27 : 63–71
12. Stricklin GP, Li L, Jancic V, Wenczak BA, Nanney LB (1993) Localization of mRNAs representing collagenase and TIMP in sections of healing human burn wounds. Am J Pathol 143 : 1657-1666
13. Saarialho-Kere UK, Chang ES, Welgus HG, Parks WC (1992) Distinct localization of collagenase and TIMP expression in wound healing associated with ulcerative pyogenic granuloma. J Clin Invest 90 : 1952–1957
14. Saarialho-Kere UK, Chang ES, Welgus HG, Parks WC (1993) Expression of interstitial collagenase, 92 kDa gelatinase, and TIMP-1 in granuloma annulare and necrobiosis lipoidica diabeticorum. J Invest Dermatol 100 : 335–342
15. Welgus HG, Stricklin GP (1983) Human skin fibroblast collagenase inhibitor: comparative studies in human connective tissues, serum and amniotic fluid. J Biol Chem 258 : 12259–12264

16. Saarialho-Kere UK, Vaalamo M, Airola K, Niemi K-M, Oikarinen AI, Parks WC (1995) Interstitial collagenase is expressed by keratinocytes which are actively involved in re-epithelialization in blistering skin diseases. J Invest Dermatol 104 : 982–988

17. Stenn KS, Malhotra R (1992) Epithelialization: In: Cohen IK, Diegelmann RF, Linblad WJ (eds) Wound healing: biochemical and clinical aspects. Saunders, Philadelphia, pp 115–127

18. Clark RAF, Lanigan JM, DellaPelle P, Manseau E, Dvorak HF, Colvin RB (1982) Fibronectin and fibrin provide a provisional matrix for epidermal cell migration during wound re-epithelization. J Invest Dermatol 79 : 264–269

19. Sudbeck PD, Parks WC, Welgus HG, Pentland AP (1994) Collagen-mediated induction of keratinocyte collagenase is mediated by tyrosine kinase and protein kinase C activities. J Biol Chem 269 : 30022–30029

20. Petersen MJ, Woodley DT, Stricklin GP, O'Keefe EJ (1990) Enhanced synthesis of collagenase by human keratinocytes cultured on type I or type IV collagen. J Invest Dermatol 94 : 341–346

21. Cavani A, Zambruno G, Marconi A, Manca V, Marchetti M, Giannetti A (1993) Distinctive integrin expression in the newly forming epidermis during wound repair. J Invest Dermatol 101 : 600–604

22. Hertle MD, Kubler M-D, Leigh IM, Watt FM (1992) Aberrant integrin expression during epidermal wound healing and in psoriatic epidermis. J Clin Invest 89 : 1892–1901

23. Juhasz I, Murphey GF, Yan H-C, Herlyn M, Albelda SM (1993) Regulation of extracellular matrix proteins and integrin cell substratum adhesion receptors on epithelium during cutaneous wound healing in vivo. Am J Pathol 143 : 1458-1469

24. Larjava H, Salo T, Haapasalmi K, Kramer RH, Heino J (1993) Expression of integrins and basement membrane components by wound keratinocytes. J Clin Invest 92 : 1425–1435

25. Staatz WD, Rajpara SM, Wayner EA, Carter WG, Santoro SA (1989) The membrane glycoprotein Ia–IIa (VLA-2) complex mediates the Mg^{+2}-dependent adhesion of platelets to collagen. J Cell Biol 108 : 1917–1924

26. Firestein GS, Paine MM, Littman BH (1991) Gene expression (collagenase, tissue inhibitor to metalloproteinases, complement, and HLA-DR) in rheumatoid arthritis and osteoarthritis synovium. Quantitative analysis and effect of intraarticular corticosteroids. Arthritis Rheum 34 : 1094–1105

27. Thompson RW, Mertens RA, Liao S, Holmes DR, Mecham RP, Welgus HG, Parks WC (1995) Production and localization of 92-kD gelatinase in abdominal aortic aneurysms: an elastolytic metalloproteinase expressed by aneurysm-infiltrating macrophages. J Clin Invest 96 : 318–327

28. Saarialho-Kere UK, Kovacs SO, Pentland AP, Parks WC, Welgus HG (1994) Distinct populations of keratinocytes express stromelysin-1 and -2 in chronic wounds. J Clin Invest 94 : 79–88

29. Bullen EC, Longaker MT, Updike DL, Benton R, Ladin D, Hou Z, Howard EW (1995) Tissue inhibitor of metalloproteinases-1 is decreased and activated gelatinases are increased in chronic wounds. J Invest Dermatol 104 : 236-240

Interview

What cytokines induce or stimulate collagenase-1 expression in keratinocytes?

Parks: A number of cytokines have been shown to affect collagenase-1 production in cultured keratinocytes. Among these, epidermal growth factor (EGF) and transforming growth factor-α (TGFα) are potent stimulators of collagenase-1 production and, especially TGFα, potentially physiologically relevant factors in cutaneous wound repair. In addition, we and others have found that collagenase-1 expression is increased in epidermal cells exposed to transforming growth factor-β (TGFβ) and γ-interferon and is repressed by basic fibroblast growth factor (bFGF). Interestingly, in other cell types, such as fibroblasts and endothelial cells, TGFβ down-regulates collagenase-1 expression and bFGF stimulates enzyme production. Thus, these two cytokines may play a role in regulating the site- and cell-specific production of MMPs in different tissue compartments and at different stages of wound repair.

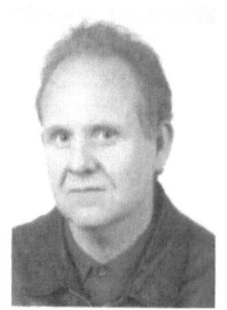

Furthermore, we do not know what cytokines would be responsible for the overproduction of collagenase-1 in chronic wounds, and actually, we really do not yet know if cytokines are responsible for aberrant MMP expression in pathologic tissue. Because cell-cell and cell-matrix interactions are quite similar between normally healing and chronic wounds, we hypothesize that some soluble factor or combination of factors contributes to persistent inflammation and an inability of the tissue to repair. Further studies are needed to identify which factors, whether intrinsic or extrinsic, lead to a chronic wound.

What is known about the induction of stromelysin expression by keratinocytes?

Parks: There are two stromelysins (-1 and -2) which are distinct gene products yet degrade the same spectrum of extracellular matrix components and with similar efficiency. These two MMPs have different regulatory elements in their promoters, suggesting that their production is regulated by different factors. Indeed, Brinkerhoff and colleagues have shown that stromelysin-1 production is stimulated by interleukin-1 and PDGF, whereas stromelysin-2 expression is largely unaffected by these agents, and that human fibroblasts produce high levels of stromelysin-1 but only negligible amounts of stromelysin-2.

In a variety of human chronic ulcers, we found that stromelysin-2 was produced in many, but not all specimens by the same keratinocytes that express collagenase-1. Stromelysin-1, on the other hand, is produced by keratinocytes in a subset of specimens, but by basal cells that are more distal to the wound edge and reside on an intact basement membrane. Often, both stromelysins were detected in the same chronic ulcer specimen, but neither was seen in normally healing wounds.

We do not yet know what influences stromelysin expression in keratinocytes, but this is an active area of investigation in our group. As stated, cell-matrix and cell-cell interactions would be similar in both chronic and acute wounds; hence, we assume that cytokines would be responsible for the aberrant production of the stromelysins in nonhealing ulcers, similar to the control of excessive collagenase-1 production in such lesions. If we can identify the soluble factors controlling expression of these MMPs, then we may discover an underlying cause of impaired healing.

What is known about the influence of topical drugs or dressings on the expression of MMPs by keratinocytes?

Parks: We do know that glucocorticoids effectively repress MMP production in a variety of cell types. Topical steroids hinder wound healing, and this is consistent with our idea that collagenase-1 is needed for epidermal repair. However, because steroids have numerous biological effects, it would be imprudent to suggest that these compounds inhibit healing simply be repressing MMP production. It is possible, though, that steroid-mediated down-regulation of MMP production may contribute to impair healing. One group of compounds which may be of particular interest in this respect is antibiotics. Tetracycline and related compounds inhibit the catalytic activity of MMPs. Although the biochemical mechanism of this inhibition is not well understood, the antibiotics apparently do not influence cellular production of MMPs. Thus, they likely act by interfering with activation, zinc coordination, substrate recognition, or catalytic activity. You may ask, then, that if collagenase-1 is needed for efficient re-epithelialization, as I hypothesize, why do wounds repair well with the application of topical antibiotics? The answer to this apparent discrepancy may be twofold. First, metalloproteinases, and collagenase-1 in particular, may not be essential for repair but rather facilitate cell migration. Second, antibiotics may create an environment that is more conducive to repair. Thus, in the absence of bacterial-induced inflammation, repair may proceed smoothly, even though MMPs are inhibited to some degree.

Inhibition of Human Neutrophil Elastase by Lipophilic Heparin and Dextran Derivatives

W. Hornebeck[1, 3], V. Bizot-Foulon[1], A. Meddahi[2], and
B. Pellat[1]

Summary

Heparin is a noncompetitive hyperbolic inhibitor of neutrophil elastase and, to a lesser extent, cathepsin G. Synthesized heparinoids with no or low anticoagulant activity, such as N-oleoyl (1, 3) heparin, inhibit neutrophil elastase and cathepsin G, interfere with urokinase and plasmin activities, and bind to elastin. Derivatized dextrans inhibit neutrophil elastase and plasmin and protect fibronectin and basic fibroblast growth factor against proteolysis. Derivatized dextrans also modulate collagen and metalloproteinase expression from human fibroblasts in culture.

Introduction

Azurophilic granules of polymorphonuclear neutrophils segregate several endopeptidases that can be secreted in active forms following cell stimulation during inflammation [1]. Human neutrophil elastase (HNE), present at millimolar concentration within these granules, exhibits a broad specificity since it can hydrolyze many extracellular matrix macromolecules (ECM) and a variety of plasma proteins [2–4].

The expression of neutral proteinases in wound healing is under the control of cytokines and growth factors; except for leukocyte proteinases – elastase, cathepsin G, and proteinase 3, endopeptidases are secreted from cells as zymogens, and a proteolytic cascade can generate active forms of matrix metalloproteinases (MMPs) involved mainly in ECM remodeling [5, 6]; impaired control of MMPs often leads to degenerative diseases [6, 7]. Figure 1 illustrates the importance of leukocyte elastase in such a proteolytic cascade and more generally in

[1] Laboratoire de Biochimie, Faculté de Chirurgie dentaire, Université René Descartes-Paris V, Montrouge, France
[2] Laboratoire CRRET, U.R.A. 1813, Université Parix XII, Créteil, France
[3] Laboratoire de Biochimie et Biologie Médicale (EP 89 CNRS), Faculté de Médicine, 51 Rue Cognacq Jay, 51095 Reims, France

Fig. 1. Importance of leukocyte elastase in extracellular matrix degradation

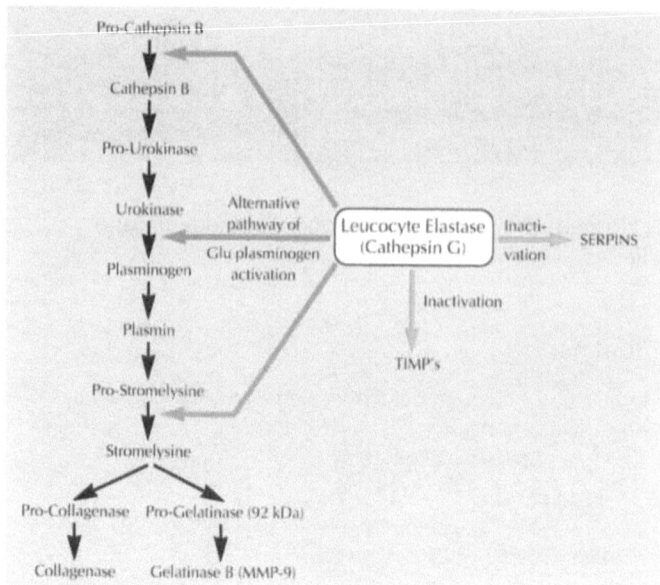

ECM catabolism. It was found to activate procathepsin B [8] and prostromelysin (MMP3) [9] and also to participate in an alternative pathway of Glu plasminogen activation [10]. In addition, it can inactivate, by proteolysis, several serine proteinase inhibitors such as antithrombin III and α2-antiplasmin, as well as tissue inhibitors of metalloproteinase [10, 11].

The contribution of HNE to human emphysematous lesions is well documented [12] and it is assumed to actively contribute to the progression of periodontal diseases [13]. It must be emphasized that periodontitis, characterized by chronic inflammatory states partly due to invading bacteria, leading to a loss of periodontal tissues, affects more than 50% of the world population over 50 years of age.

The crevicular fluid of patients suffering from periodontitis contains high levels of neutral protease activities which can be reduced significantly following basic periodontal treatment [14]. Recent investigations demonstrated that within the crevicular fluid of periodontitis patients, neutrophil elastase could be determined both in its complex form with α1-proteinase inhibitor and in its free form [15]; these data indicated that the levels of free enzyme exceed those of its main natural inhibitor. Impaired α1-Pi functionality could result from either oxidation of a critical methionine residue in its active site or its degradation by other proteinases [16]. It was also shown that the quantities of free elastase in crevicular fluid of patients with rapid periodontitis were correlated with probing depth and attachment loss: 0.074 nM ± 0.037 in the 4- to 5-mm depth group as compared with 0.206 nM ± 0.057 in the 6- to 7-mm group. The levels of active collagenase and gelatinase are also exacerbated in the crevicular fluid of patients with periodontal disease; interestingly, in oral rinse samples of patients, gelatinase and elastase activities were correlated, suggesting a potential in vivo activation of the MMP cascade by elastase [16].

The antielastase control system comprises four proteinaceous inhibitors: α2-macroglobulin, α1-proteinase inhibitor, mucus proteinase inhibitor, and elafin [17, 18]. Supplementation with exogenous inhibitors is regarded the main pharmacological route to shift the proteinase-antiproteinase imbalance. The use of high-molecular-weight protease inhibitors, which can be produced by recombinant technology, was considered as the first approach [19]. Another strategy consists in the design and development of low-molecular-weight synthetic elastase inhibitors. Such substances might present several advantages over large protein molecules in terms of rates of absorption, enzyme selectivity, and lowered risk of immunological response [20].

Taking into account the neutrophil elastase characteristic of binding tightly to both polyanions and hydrophobic compounds, we developed a novel class of elastase inhibitors: lipophilic heparin or dextran derivatives.

Interaction Between Heparin and Neutrophil Elastase

The polypeptide chain of neutrophil elastase comprises two structurally similar antiparallel β barrel cylindrical domains, and its active site triad Ser 195 – His 57 is localized within the crevice between these two domains. Such a structure is shared by most class-I serine proteinases. Neutrophil elastase is a very basic molecule (pI ≈ 10), due to the presence of 19 arginines balanced by only nine acidic residues, three of which are buried inside the molecule [21]. In several aspects, proteinases from polymorphonuclear azurophilic granules resemble chymases concentrated in mast cell secretory granules [22]. Several of these proteinases, such as MCP4a5, are sequestered within cell granules as complexes with heparan-sulfate proteoglycans; since such binding did not affect enzyme activity, it was hypothesized that it might impede enzyme autolysis or shield it against inactivation by circulating natural proteinase inhibitors.

In keeping with such analogy, we explored the putative binding of heparin to HNE and its influence on enzyme activity.

Table 1. Heparin-binding consensus sequences

A Heparin-binding consensus amino acid sequence [22]. *B* refers to a basic amino acid [mainly Arg *(R)*] and *X* to any other

Amino acid consensus sequence (Heparin binding)	X.<u>B.B.</u>X.B.X.
	X.B.B.B.X.X.B.X
Leukocyte elastase	G.<u>R.R.</u>A.R.P
	4 5 6 7 8 9

B Inhibition of human neutrophil elastase by heparin and tetrasaccharide fragments

	Ki (nM)
Heparin	70×10^{-6}
Tetrasaccharides	
Series I	100
Series II	76
Series III	16×7

In contrast to mast cell chymases, heparin binding to HNE reduced proteinase activity. Enzyme inhibition was classified as hyperbolic and noncompetitive with Ki = 75 nM assuming Mr (heparin) $\approx$ 12 000 [23, 24].

Heparin and heparan sulfate interact with many proteins, and such binding interferes with several important biological functions: coagulation, lipoprotein metabolism, and cell growth [25, 26]. The concept of interactive specificity between polypeptide and glycosaminoglycan chains is gradually emerging [27]. From the polypeptide side, heparin-binding consensus sequences have been delineated (Table 1A). Such a hypothesis needs to be modified, since several proteins, e.g., FGF-2, do not contain such a consensus sequence; furthermore, the important amino acids comprising the heparin-binding domain may be located in different peptide loops of the molecule. Nevertheless, HNE does contain such a heparin-binding sequence in its N-terminal moiety (Table 1A).

It was postulated that the occurrence of two arginine residues located 2 nm apart and separated by either α-helical or β-strand polypeptide might be of primordial importance for heparin binding [27]. As pinpointed by Bode et al. [28], all but two of the HNE arginines are located in patches on the surface of the enzyme, whereas the side chains of Arg 217 and Arg 117 are situated near the active site of the proteinase. Arg 217 was considered an important determinant in P4–S4 interactions between HNE and the substrate, and formation of an ion pair with such a residue often led to reduction of enzyme activity. This might imply that heparin binding to HNE involved some cooperation between the above-mentioned consensus sequence and Arg 217.

Although most protein-glycosaminoglycan interactions were originally considered nonspecific, involving purely electrostatic interactions, the general idea of specific GAG sequences recognizing defined protein sequences is now in fashion. Such a concept originates from the pioneer investigations of Choay and colleagues aiming to characterize antithrombin III-heparin interactions and from the discovery of an unusual pentasaccharide in the glycosaminoglycan molecule [29]. Since then, a defined oligosaccharide sequence recognizing FGF-2 has been identified [30], and similar searches for other chemokines are under way. It has to be mentioned that such specificity also underlines the notion of conformational flexibility of IdoUA-containing GAGs, as pointed out by Casu and colleagues [31]. Particularly OSO_3^- seemed to influence mainly the conformation of this saccharide toward a more reactive structure. It needs to be underlined that at a similar extent of sulfation, OSO_3^- tetrasaccharides are better HNE inhibitors than N-sulfated molecules (Table 1B).

Lipophilic Heparin and Dextran Derivatives as Neutrophil Elastase Inhibitors

In contrast to most serine proteinases, neutrophil elastase displays a broad specificity and, besides elastin, can degrade a wide range of hydrophobic molecules [2, 3]. This property is probably related to the presence of an extended hydrophobic binding site located in the vicinity of its active site. This hydrophobic binding pocket can accommodate a variety of ligands with very different structures. Long-chain *cis* (but not *trans*) unsaturated fatty acids and peptide derivatives were first reported to inhibit HNE [32, 33]. As shown by Tyagi and Simon [34], the interaction of oleic acid with the enzyme was characterized by two apparent inhibitory modes: a high-affinity one with Ki = 48 ± 3 µM, resulting in partial noncompetitive inhibltion, and a competitive inhibitory mode of lower affinity with Ki = 16 ± 1 nM [34]. In this latter mode of binding, the participation of a positively charged residue, Arg ± 217, located in the P4 subsite of HNE was evidenced [34]. *cis*-Parinaric acid, derived from the plant *Parinary laurinium* behaves similarly to oleic acid [35], and neutrophil elastase is also inhibited by ursolic acid, a pentacyclic triterpenoid present in

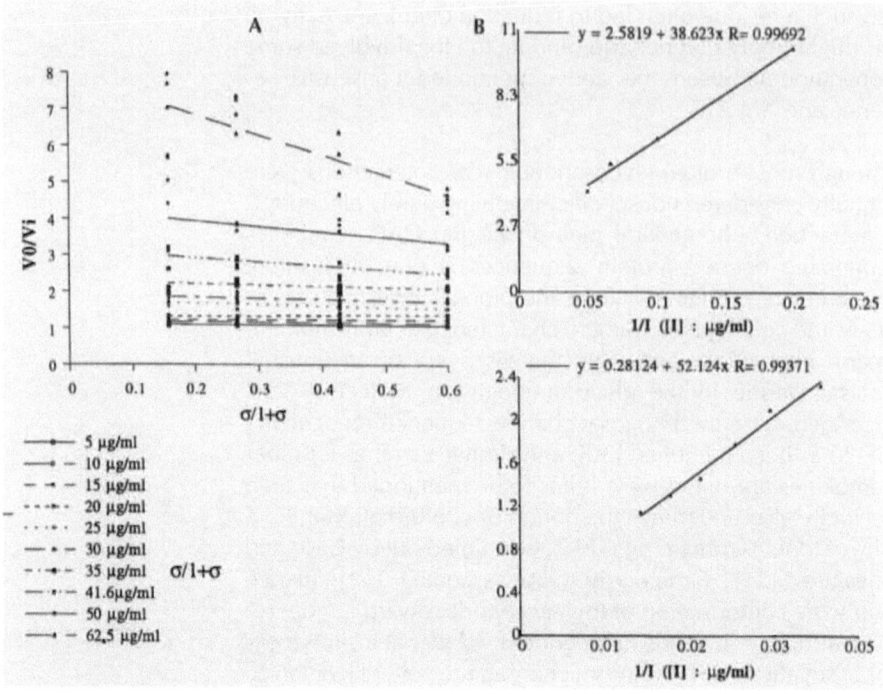

Fig. 2 A, B. Inhibition of HNE by CER: specific velocity plot and Kis. Five to 62.5 μg/ml of CER were incubated for 5 min at 37.0 ± 0.1° C in the presence of HNE (E0 = 16.1 nM) in 100 mM Tris-HCl, pH 8.0, containing 0.01% Triton X-100 (v/v) and 0.02% NaN3 (w/v), before adding MeOSucAlaAlaProValNA (0.025–0.2 mM); release of paranitroanilide was recorded at 410 nm. **A** specific velocity plot: σ = [S]/Km at ten concentrations of CER. **B** Kis were determined by the replot of the intercepts with y-axis (a) versus the inverse of the inhibitor concentration ([I] expressed in μg/ml)

great abundance in the wax-like coating of apples and several other fruits [36].

We have recently turned our attention to ceramides and to isolating such substances from wheat. Apart from maintaining proper skin functions, ceramides can influence cell growth and differentiation and may also mediate apoptosis in HL-60 leukemia cells [37]. Wheat ceramides composed of dehydro-phytosphingosine, phytosphingosine, and polyunsaturated fatty acids were tested for their ability to interfere with HNE activity [38]. The main nonhydroxylated fatty acids were palmitic acids (16:0), oleic acid (18:1), and linoleic acid (18:2), which accounted, respectively, for 19, 12, and 53% of total fatty acids. Either ceramides (CER) or glycosyl ceramides (gly-CER) were found to react very fast (in a few seconds) with HNE. Kinetic data were analyzed by the specific velocity plot representation. For CER, the plot consisted, at low ceramide concentrations (< 20 μg/ml), in a family of parallel lines (Fig. 2). Increasing CER concentrations led to deviations of parallelism. Therefore, at low concentrations, HNE inhibition can be classified as hyperbolic noncompetitive. For higher concentrations of ceramides, inhibition became linearly mixed. The same inhibition mode was observed for glyCER. Linearization by replots of a = a–1 versus inverse inhibitor concentration

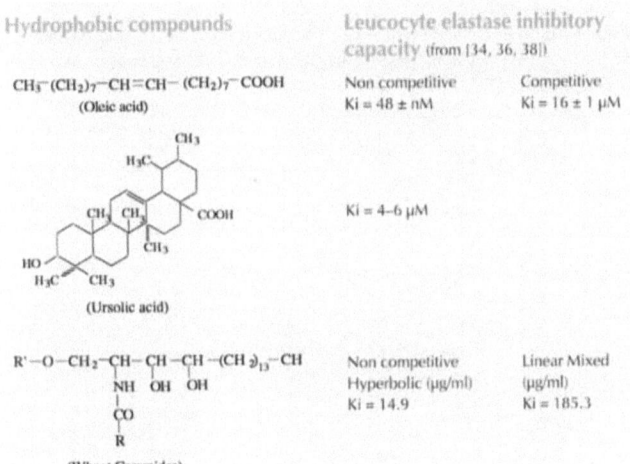

Hydrophobic compounds | Leucocyte elastase inhibitory capacity (from [34, 36, 38])

CH₃-(CH₂)₇-CH=CH-(CH₂)₇-COOH
(Oleic acid)

Non competitive
Ki = 48 ± nM

Competitive
Ki = 16 ± 1 µM

(Ursolic acid)

Ki = 4–6 µM

R'—O—CH₂—CH—CH—CH—(CH₂)₁₃—CH
        | | |
        NH   OH   OH
        |
        CO
        |
        R

(Wheat Ceramides)

Non competitive
Hyperbolic (µg/ml)
Ki = 14.9

Linear Mixed
(µg/ml)
Ki = 185.3

Fig. 3. Inhibition of leukocyte elastase by hydrophobic natural substances

(Fig. 2 and legend) allowed us to determine Kis corresponding to noncompetitive and mixed inhibitions (Fig. 3).

The simultaneous presence of a heparin-binding site and a hydrophobic pocket, both of which reduced HNE activity, prompted us to synthesize lipophilic heparin derivatives with the hope of improving the elastase inhibitory capacity of the individual counterparts [24, 39]. N-oleoyl-heparin derivatives (with no anticoagulant activity) differing in their oleic acid and sulfate contents were synthesized and studied for their abilities to inhibit neutrophil elastase and cathepsin G (Table 2). The covalent coupling of oleic acid to heparin did not modify the nature of enzyme inhibitions, since the main driving force for the interaction between enzymes and glycosaminoglycans was electrostatic, and inhibitions for all compounds were classified as tight-binding hyperbolic and noncompetitive. Introducing one oleic acid residue per three disaccharide units of partially N-desulfated heparin lowered enzyme inhibition and the stoichiometry of binding as compared with heparin. Re-N-sulfatation of N-oleoyl-heparin derivative to SO_3^-/COO^- values similar to those for heparin restored both inhibitory capacity and the stoichiometry of binding. Therefore, our initial attempt to design elastase inhibitors of higher potency by coupling unsaturated fatty acids to heparin was rather unsuccessful. However, in contrast to individual parent molecules, N-oleoyl heparin derivatives did suppress the activity of several serine proteinases: porcine pancreatic elastase, plasmin, urokinase, and α-chymotrypsin [39].

Anionic polymers other than heparins, such as pentosan polysulfate [40] and MDL [41] (see formula, Fig. 4), were shown to

Table 2. Kinetic parameters for inhibition of human neutrophil elastase (HNE) and cathepsin G (CatG) by heparin and two oleylated heparins (Ol1 : 3Hep and Ol1 : 5Hep (SO4) from [24])

	HNE	CatG
Heparin		
K_i	0.9 ± 0.5 (0.075)	< 0.3 (< 0.025)
β	0.15 ± 0.02	0.40 ± 0.02
Stoichiometry	2.08	4.3
Ol1 : Hep		
K_i	3.6 ± 1.3 (0.3)	115 ± 40 (9.5)
β	0.16 ± 0.01	0.09 ± 0.02
Stoichiometry	1.06	2.6
Ol1 : 5Hep(SO$_4$)		
K_i	0.15 ± 0.01	0.19 ± 0.02
β	0.15 ± 0.01	0.19 ± 0.02
Stoichiometry	2.7	2.4

inhibit HNE. Dextrans are polymers of D-glucopyranose produced by *Lactobacillus casei* in which a majority of sugar units are linked as α [1–6]. Such a link might provide a flexible conformational frame for the polymer to which functionalized groups could be linked. Carboxymethyl, benzylamide, and benzylamide sulfonate, at various concentrations, were coupled to the polysaccharide backbone in order to obtain compounds displaying several interactions and properties similar to those of heparin and heparinoids. To summarize, such derivatized dextrans mimicked several biological properties of heparin, modulating cell growth [42] and acting as stabilizers, potentiators, and protectors of fibroblast growth factors [43]. We recently explored the capacity of these heparinoids to inhibit HNE. Like all anionic polymers, derivatized dextrans containing carboxymethyl and benzylamide sulfonate groups bind to this endopeptidase via electrostatic interactions and form tight complexes. Also, similar to heparin and its lipophilic derivatives, the HNE inhibition by derivatized dextrans was classified as hyperbolic and noncompetitive. Other analogies include dependency of the inhibition on the molecular weight and degree of substitution of the polymer with negatively charged benzylamide sulfonate groups (Fig. 4). Derivatized dextrans also share with N-oleoyl heparins the capacity to inhibit plasmin activity [44].

Concluding Remarks

On the basis of the dual properties of neutrophil elastase to interact with several lipophilic substances and anionic polymers, N-oleoyl heparins and dextrans derivatized with car-

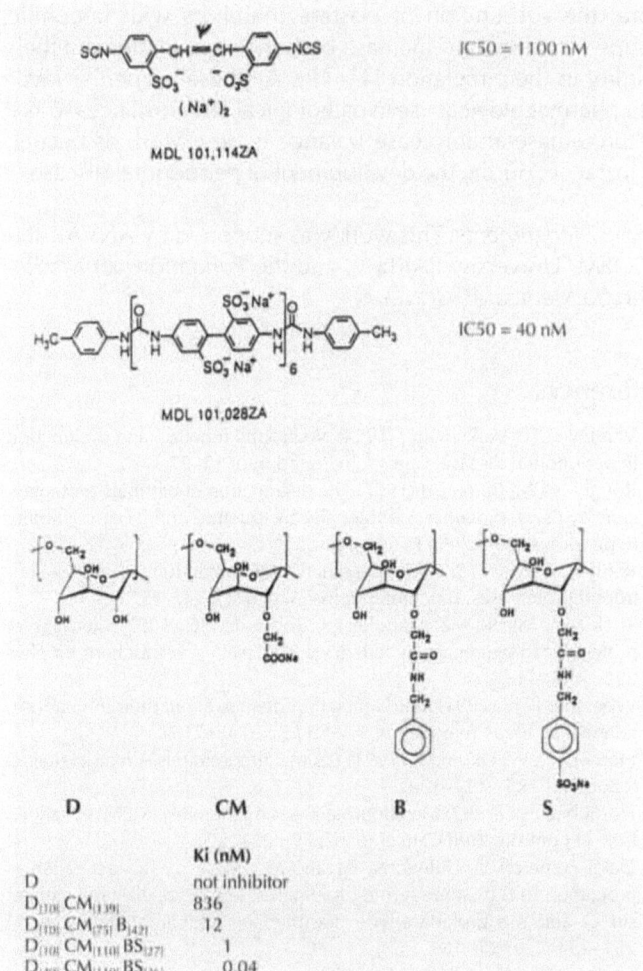

Fig. 4. Inhibition of neutrophil elastase by anionic polymers. *IC50*, Concentration of substance leading to 5% inhibition of enzyme activity; *D*, dextran; *CM*, carboxymethyl; *B*, benzylamide; *S*, sulfonate

boxymethyl and benzylamide sulfonate groups were evaluated for their inhibitory capacity toward this endopeptidase. Both types of compounds behave as tightly binding hyperbolic noncompetitive inhibitors of neutrophil elastase, with their Ki averaging those of heparin, e.g., 75 nM. However, they present several advantages compared with heparin, such as being devoid of anticoagulant acitivity and inhibiting other neutral serine proteinases, urokinase and plasmin, also actively involved in the proteolytic cascade leading to the formation of active matrix metalloproteinases. They can also modulate MMP expression either indirectly, by protecting growth factors FGFs and TNFα against proteolysis catalyzed by serine proteinases [44], or, like heparin, directly, by inhibiting enzyme gene induction by phorbol esters or interleukin 1β [45, 46]. Furthermore, the substitution of elastase inhibitors with lipophilic groups was shown to increase both their specificity and their stability in the circulation [47–49]. All these properties favor their pharmacological use in pathological circumstances where the proteinase-antiprotease balance is destroyed, as occurs, for instance, during the development of periodontal disease.

Acknowledgements. This work was supported by ANVAR-IN-OCOSM, University PARIS V, and the *Fondation pour la Recherche Médicale* (F.R.M.).

References

1. Van Dyke TE, Vaikuntam J (1994) Neutrophil function and dysfunction in periodontal disease. Curr Opin Periodontol 19–27
2. Roughley PM, Barrett AJ (1977) The degradation of cartilage proteoglycans by tissue proteinases. Proteoglycan structure and its susceptibility to proteolysis. Biochem J 167 : 629-637
3. Reilly C, Travis J (1978) The degradation of human lung elastin by neutrophil proteinases. Biochim Biophys Acta 621 : 147-157
4. Tuck Mak M, Ilic MZ, Handley CJ, Robinson HC (1992) Cleavage of proteoglycan aggregate by leucocyte elastase. Arch Biochem Biophys 292 : 442–447
5. Woessner JF JR (1991) Matrix metalloproteinases and their inhibitors in connective tissue remodeling. FASEB J 5 : 2145–2154
6. Hornebeck W, Lafuma C (1991) Les metalloproteinases matricielles. C R Soc Biol 185 : 127–134
7. Hornebeck W (1992) Metalloproteinases matricielles (MPM) et cancer. Role et contrôle. Bull Cancer (Paris) 79 : 221–225
8. Dalet-Fumeron V, Guinec N, Pagano M (1993) In vitro activation of procathepsin B by three serine-proteinases: leukocyte elastase, cathepsin G and the urokinase-type plasminogen activator. FEBS Lett 3 : 251–254
9. Nagase H, Enghild JJ, Suzuki K, Salvesen G (1990) Stepwise activation of the precursor of matrix metalloproteinase 3 (stromelysin) by proteinases and (4-aminophenyl) mercuric acetate. Biochemistry 29 : 5783–5789
10. Machovich R, Owen WG (1979) An elastase-dependent pathway of plasminogen activation. Biochemistry 28 : 4517-4522
11. Jordan RE, Nelson RM, Kilpatrick J, Newgren JO, Esmon PC, Fournel MA (1989) Inactivation of human antithrombin by neutrophil elastase. J Biol Chem 264 : 10493–10500
12. Janoff A (1985) Elastase and emphysema: current assessment of the protease-antiprotease hypothesis. Am Rev Respir Dis 132 : 417–433
13. Armitage GC, Jeffcoat MK, Chadwick DE, Taggart EJ, Numabe Y, Landis JR, Weaver SL, Sharp TJ (1994) Longitudinal evaluation of elastase as a marker for the progression of periodontitis. J Periodontol 65 : 120-128
14. Eley BM, Cox SW (1992) Cathepsin B/L, elastase, tryptase, trypsin and dipeptidyl peptidase IV-like activities in gingival crevicular fluid. A comparison of levels before and after periodontal surgery in chronic periodontitis patients. J Periodontol 63 : 412-417
15. Guessous F, Huynh C, Godeau G, Giroud JP, Meyer J, Roch-Arveiller M (1995) Active and α1-proteinase inhibitor complexed leukocyte elas-

tase levels in crevicular fluids from patients with periodontal diseases. Int J Pharmacol (submitted)

16. Makela M, Salö T, Uitto VJ, Larjava H (1994) Matrixmetalloproteinases (MMP2 and MMP9) of the oral cavity: cellular origin and relationship to periodontal status. J Dent Res 73 : 1397–1406

17. Cawell RW (1990) The molecular structure and pathology of α1-antitrypsin. Lung [Suppl] Carrell 530-534

18. Qi-Long Ying, Simon SR (1993) Kinetics of the inhibition of human leukocyte elastase by elafin, a 6-kilodalton elastase-specific inhibitor (mutant and the effects of these mutations on secretion of the variant inhibitors. J Biol Chem 266 : 7578–7582

19. McCracken AA, Kruse KB, Valentine J, Roberts C, Yohannes TZ, Brown JL (1991) Construction and expression of α1-proteinase inhibitor mutants and the effects of these mutations on secretion of the variant inhibitors. J Biol Chem 266 : 7578–7582

20. Edwards PD, Bernstein PR (1994) Synthetic inhibitors of elastase. Med Res Rev 14 : 127-194

21. Naria MA, McKeever BM, Springer JP, Leu Yin T, Williams MR, Fluder EM, Dorn CP, Hoogsteen K (1989) Structure of human neutrophil elastase in complex with a peptide chlorometry ketone inhibitor at 1.84 A resolution. Proc Natl Acad Sci USA 86 : 7-11

22. Sali A, Matnimoto R, McNeil MP, Karplus M, Stevens RL (1993) Three-dimensional models of four mast cell chymases. J Biol Chem 268 : 9023–9034

23. Redini F, Tixier JM, Petitou M, Choay J, Robert L, Hornebeck W (1988) Inhibition of leukocyte elastase by heparin and its derivatives. Biochem J 252 : 515-519

24. Baici A, Diezhazi C, Neszmehzi A, Moczar E, Hornebeck W (1993) Inhibition of the human leukocyte endopeptidase elastase and cathepsin G and of porcine pancreatic elastase by N-oleoyl derivatives of heparin. Biochem Pharmacol 46 : 1545–1549

25. Maccarama M, Casu B, Lindhahl U (1993) Minimal sequence in heparin-heparan sulphate required for binding of basic fibroblast growth factor. J Biol Chem 268 : 23898-23905

26. San Antonio JD, Sloven J, Lawler J, Karnovsky MJ, Lander AD (1993) Specificity in the interactions of extracellular matrix proteins with subpopulations of the glycosaminiglycan heparin. Biochemistry 32 : 4746–4756

27. Spillmann D, Lindahl H (1994) Glycosaminoglycan-protein interactions: a question of specificity. Curr Opin Struct Biol 4 : 667–682

28. Bode W, Meyer E, Powers JC (1989) Human leukocyte and porcine pancreatic elastase: X-ray crystal structures, mechanism, substrate specificity and mechanism-based inhibitors. Biochemistry 28 : 1951–1963

29. Atha DH, Lormeau JC, Petitou M, Rosenberg RD, Choay J (1985) Contribution of monosaccharide residues in heparin binding to antithrombin III. Biochemistry 24 : 6723–6729

30. Maccarama M, Casu B, Lindahl U (1993) Minimal sequence in heparin-heparan sulphate required for binding of basic fibroblast growth factor. J Biol Chem 260 : 23898-23905

31. Casu B, Petitou M, Provasoli M, Sinaÿ P (1988) Conformational flexibility: a new concept for explaining binding and biological properties of iduronic acid containing glycosaminoglycans. TIBS 13 : 221–225

32. Ashe BM, Zimmerman H (1977) Ashe BM, Zimmerman H (1977) Specific inhibition of human granulocyte elastase by cis-unsaturated fatty acids and activation by the corresponding alcohols. Biochem Biophys Res Commun 75 : 194-199

33. Hornebeck W, Moczar E, Szecsi J, Robert L (1985) Fatty acid peptide derivatives as model compounds to protect elastin against degradation by elastases. Biochem Pharmacol 34 : 3315–3321

34. Tyagi SC, Simon SR (1991) Parinaric acids as probes of binding domains in neutrophil elastase. J Biol Chem 266 : 15105–15191

35. Ying QL, Rinehart AR, Simon SR, Cherouis JC (1991) Inhibition of human leucocyte elastase by ursolic acid. Biochem J 277 : 521–526

36. Simonsen J, Ross WCJ (1957) The terpenes, vol. 5. Cambridge University Press, Cambridge, pp 114-135

37. Hannun YA, Obeid LM (1995) Ceramide, an intracellular signal for apoptosis. TIBS 20 : 73–77

38. Bizot-Foulon V, Guessous F, Lati G, Rousset G, Roch-Arveiller M, Hornebeck W (1995) Inhibition of human neutrophil elastase by wheat ceramides. Int J Cosm Sci (in press)

39. Hornebeck W, Lafuma C, Robert L, Moczar M, Moczar E (1994) Heparin and its derivatives modulate serine proteinases (serpro)-serine proteinase inhibitors (serpins) balance. Pathol Res Pract 190 : 895–902

40. Baici A, Salgman P, Feler K, Boui A (1984) Inhibition of human elastase from polymorphonuclear leukocytes by gold sodium thiomalate and pentosan polysuolphonate (SP-54). Biochem Pharmacol 30 : 703–708

41. Janusz MJ, Mare M (1994) Inhibition of human neutrophil elastase and cathepsin G by a biphenyl disulphonic acid copolymer. Int J Immunopharmacol 16 : 623–632

42. Bagheri-Yarmand, Bittoun P, Champion J, Letourneur D, Jozefonvicz J, Fernadjian S, Crepin M (1994) Carboxymethyl benzylamide dextrans inhibit breast cell growth. Dev Biol 30A : 822–824

43. Tardieu M, Gamby C, Avramoglou T, Jozefonvicz J, Barritault D (1992) Derivatized dextrans mimic heparin as stabilizers, potentiators and protectors of acidic or basic FGF. J Cell Physiol 150 : 194–203

44. Meddahi A, Lemdjabar H, Caruelle JP, Barritault D, Hornebeck W (1995) Inhibition by dextran derivatives of FGF-2 plasmin mediated degradation. Biochimie (in press)

45. Kitamura, Maruyama N, Mitowai T, Yokoo T, Sakai O (1994) Heparin selectively inhibits gene expressin of matrix metalloproteinase transit in cultured mesangial cells. Biochem Biophys Res Commun 203 : 1335-1338

46. Kenagy RD, Nikkarsi ST, Welgus HG, Clowes AW (1994) Heparin inhibits the induction of three matrix metalloproteinases (stromelysin, 92 kDa gelatinases and collagenase) in primate arterial smooth muscle cells. J Clin Invest 93 : 1987–1993

47. Kerneur C, Hornebeck W, Robert L, Moczar L (1993) Inhibition of human leucocyte elastase by fatty acyl benzisothiazolinone, 1,1-dioxide conjugates. Biochem Pharmacol 45 : 1889-1895

48. Hlasta DJ, Bell MR, Court JJ, Fundy KC, Desai RC, Ferguson EW, Gordon RJ, Kumar V, Maycock AL, Subramanyyam C (1995) The design of potent and stable benzisothiazolinone inhibitors of human leucocyte elastase. Bioorg Med Chem 5 : 331–336

49. Salvin S, Petitou M, Lormeau JC, Dupouy D, Sie P, Caranobe C, Hovin G, Bonen B (1992) Pharmacologic properties of an unfractionated heparin butyryl derivative with long-lasting effects. J Lab Clin Med 119 : 189–196

Interview

What could be a potential therapeutic consequence of your research?

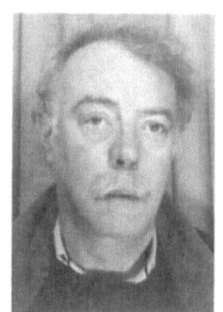

Hornebeck: Human neutrophil elastase is involved in the pathogenesis of emphysema, rheumatoid arthritis, periodontitis, and several inflammatory disorders. Lipophilic heparin or dextran derivatives are extremely potent inhibitors of this enzyme and therefore could be of therapeutic value in these diseases. More generally, by acting as stabilizers, potentiators of growth factors, they can accelerate matrix remodeling following injury. This has been demonstrated in several wound-healing models (skin, bone, muscle).

Do the investigated heparinoids act comparably in a chronic wound?

Hornebeck: The influence of heparinoids was not investigated in a chronic wound.

Is anything known about the penetration of these heparinoids into the wound after topical application?

Hornebeck: Dextran derivatized with carboxymethyl benzylamide sulfonate groups was labeled with ([4,6-dichlorotriazine-2yl] amino) fluorescein and applied topically to the skin of harlen rats at the wounded area. On day 1 following application, labeled dextran was identified within the epidermis and maximally at the margin of the scar.

Chemotactic Properties of Human Collagen Breakdown Products in Wound Healing

M. Radice, L. Cardarelli, R. Cortivo, and G. Abatangelo

Summary

During wound healing, cells are attracted by many stimuli to the injured area. Many substances are known to have a chemotactic effect on different cells. Among those, human collagen breakdown products (HCBP) have been shown to be chemotactic in vitro for fibroblasts and white blood cells. In our experiments, collagen (types I and III) extracted from the human placenta was enzymatically digested with bacterial collagenase (Knoll AG, Germany). Breakdown peptides were then used both in vitro and in vivo to evaluate their proliferative and chemotactic activities. HCBP were demonstrated to have a proliferative effect on murine and human fibroblasts, while they showed a chemotactic effect in a model of wound healing in the rat.

Introduction

Wound healing is a complex process necessary for every organism to defend itself from external and internal injuries. A network of several elements, such as distinct cell populations, growth factors, cytokines, enzymes, and ECM molecules, forms to restore the wounded area. With regard to adult mammals, the entire process is generally divided into different, partly overlapping phases: clot formation and inflammation, granulation tissue formation, angiogenesis, and tissue remodeling.

During the early phase of inflammation the organization of an immune response which will face a potential lethal infection is very important. Initially, polymorphonuclear leukocytes (PMNs) infiltrate the site of the injury, constituting the first defensive barrier. Subsequently, the monocyte/macrophage presence is essential in order to resolve the inflammation and start the formation of granulation tissue. In particular, these

---

Institute of Histology, Faculty of Medicine, University of Padua, Italy

phagocytes provide an active tissue débridement and a massive signal release toward other cells such as fibroblasts, endothelial cells, and epithelial cells.

Thus the recruitment of PMNs and monocyte/macrophages is of great importance in wound healing. Many stimuli are known to be chemotactic for these cells, such as complement fragments, bacterial-derived products, cytokines, and even collagen molecules and their derived peptides. The chemotactic activity of the latter two was demonstrated in vitro [1–6]. In addition, human collagen breakdown products (HCBP) were reported to activate macrophages [7, 8] and to exert other biological activities [9, 10].

Despite this literature, few experiments on the subject have been conducted in vivo [5, 11]. The aim of our work was to assay the human collagen-derived peptides for a proliferative effect in vitro and for a chemotactic effect in vivo in a wound-repair model.

Materials and Methods

The HCBP were obtained from human placental tissue by enzymatic digestion with clostridial collagenase obtained from Knoll AG, Germany [12]. Human placental collagen was obtained as follows: immediately after delivery the placenta was washed with water and then cut into small pieces. After several washings the placental tissue was isolated with acetic acid, filtered on gauze, and then homogenized. Extraction was carried out with pepsin digestion, followed by precipitation with NaCl. After centrifugation, the pellet was suspended in Tris-HCl and dialyzed against acetic acid. The solution containing the extracted collagen was finally lyophilized and weighed.

Aliquots of purified human collagen were incubated with bacterial collagenase at an enzyme/substrate ratio of 8 : 1000 at 37° C for 90 min in Tris-HCl + $CaCl_2$ buffer, pH 7.8. The digested material was then ultrafiltered using N_2 on PM10 Amicon (Beverly, Mass.) membranes in order to separate collagenase from the breakdown products. To evaluate the efficiency of the digestion, the concentration of the collagen peptides was determined by the hydroxyproline assay [13].

In vitro and in vivo research protocols were performed. The in vitro study was conducted to verify the possibility that HCBP stimulate the growth and biosynthesis of cells. Murine (Balb/c

3T3) and human (conjunctival) fibroblasts were cultured in DMEM supplemented with either 0.4% or 10% fetal calf serum (FCS) and inoculated once with HCBP at different concentrations (range: 0.01 ng/ml⁻¹ mg/ml). The proliferation rate was measured by a simple and sensitive test [14] at three different time points: 24, 48, and 72 h for murine, and 2, 4, and 7 days for human fibroblasts; biosynthetic activity was assessed by the radiolabeling procedure (^{3}H-proline).

In order to detect a chemotactic effect of HCBP in vivo, we decided to use an animal model of wound healing. In our study, we implanted four polyvinyl alcohol sponge discs in the subcutaneous abdomen space of adult white rats (250–300 g). Sponges were afterwards injected pairwise with the substances under investigation and the negative control (normal saline solution).

Two series of experiments were done, and 18 animals were used: HCBP (1 mg) and normal saline were injected in nine, whereas clostridial collagenase (5 µg) and normal saline were injected in the remaining nine rats. Since both HCBP and bacterial collagenase are easily resorbable, we resuspended the substances in a gelatinous vehicle (2% methylcellulose).

Animals were killed at three different time points (3, 5, and 7 days postsurgery) and sponges were harvested, weighed, and processed for biochemical and histological analyses. Each specimen was cut into three parts: one half was used to determine the protein [15], DNA [16], and collagen contents [13]. The remaining two parts were either frozen or paraffin embedded. Paraffin sections were processed for hematoxylin/eosin and chloroacetate esterase [17] stainings, whereas frozen sections were used for the immunohistochemical detection of activated macrophages with ED2 (Serotec, Oxford, UK) anti-rat monoclonal antibody [17].

Results

Several series of experiments were done on fibroblast cultures. HCBP increased the proliferation rate on rat cells within a broad range of 1–1000 ng/ml. This effect was observed during all three time points considered.

Human conjunctival fibroblasts were similarly stimulated by HCBP, although a specific range of action was not determined. In Fig. 1 one such representative experiment is plotted. At day 2 no apparent effects were seen, while at day 4 cells in-

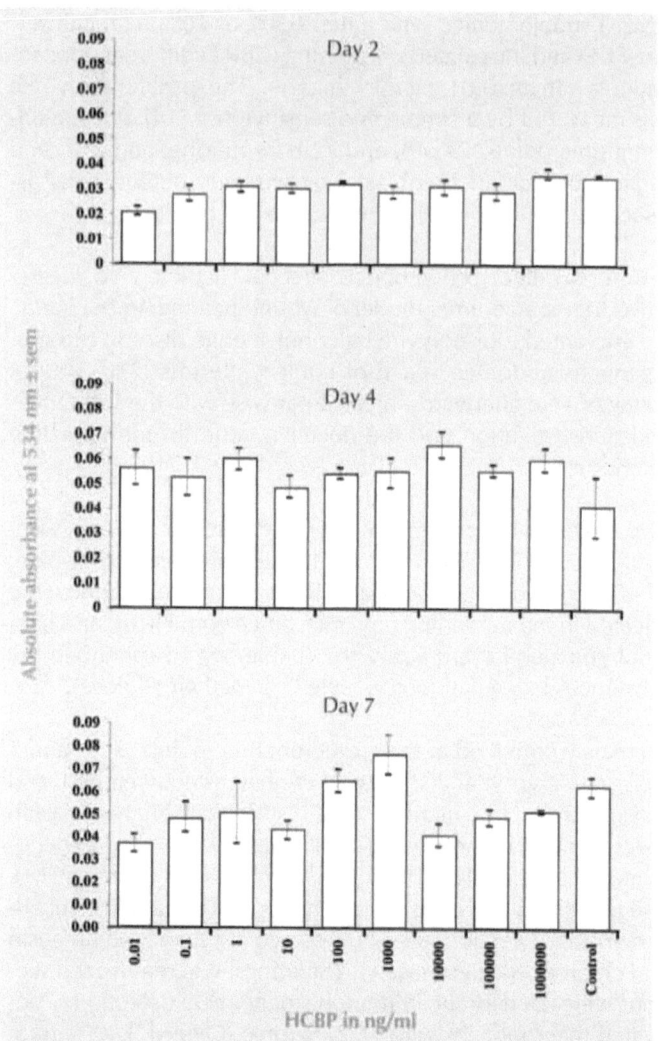

Fig. 1. HCBP proliferative effect on human fibroblasts. Cells were seeded at 2000 cells well in a 96-wells/plate cluster and cultured in DMEM supplemented with 10% FCS for 2, 4, and 7 days. Data are expressed as absolute absorbance at 534 nm ± SEM

oculated with HCBP proliferated, and reached the confluence faster (day 7) than the control. When DMEM with a low serum content (0.4%) was used, HCBP at higher concentrations (0.1–1 mg/ml) seemed to allow the human fibroblasts to maintain their growth ability (data not shown).

With regard to the biosynthesis, it seems that HCBP do not affect this cellular aspect, since results were contradictory (data not shown).

Sponges injected with HCBP demonstrated first that peptides were highly resorbable, since in 24 h they were completely dissolved in wound fluid. Nevertheless, biochemical analyses

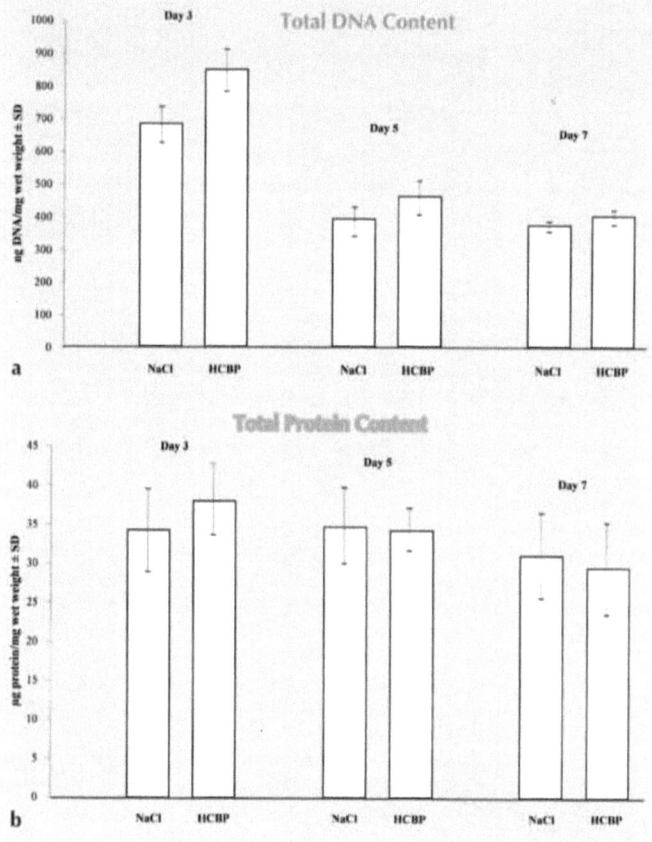

Fig. 2. DNA and protein content of rat implanted sponges. **a** DNA profile of day 3, 5, and 7 post surgery. Data are expressed as nanograms total DNA/milligram wet weight of the sponge ± SD; **b** Protein profiles of days 3, 5, and 7 post surgery. Data are expressed as micrograms total protein/milligram wet weight of the sponge ± SD

showed that HCBP injection caused an increase in the cellularity (Fig. 2) and protein content of the sponge within the first days (3–5 days post surgery) compared with the controls. The collagen content seemed to follow the same trend, but at day 7 HCBP reduced its biosynthesis. Interestingly, collagenase injection seemed to regularly increase the collagen production. Histological sections stained with hematoxylin/eosin substantially confirmed the biochemical findings, since from semi-quantitative analyses more cells were present within the sponges treated with HCBP (Fig. 3).

When we looked at the PMN infiltration using the chloroacetate esterase technique, we were also able to count a higher number of cells within the HCBP-treated samples compared with the controls (Fig. 4). Finally, macrophage infiltration was evident at day 5 and increased at day 7, as seen from the immunohistochemical staining (Fig. 5). From a semi-quantitative analysis it seemed that more macrophages were present within the HCBP-treated sponges than in the controls.

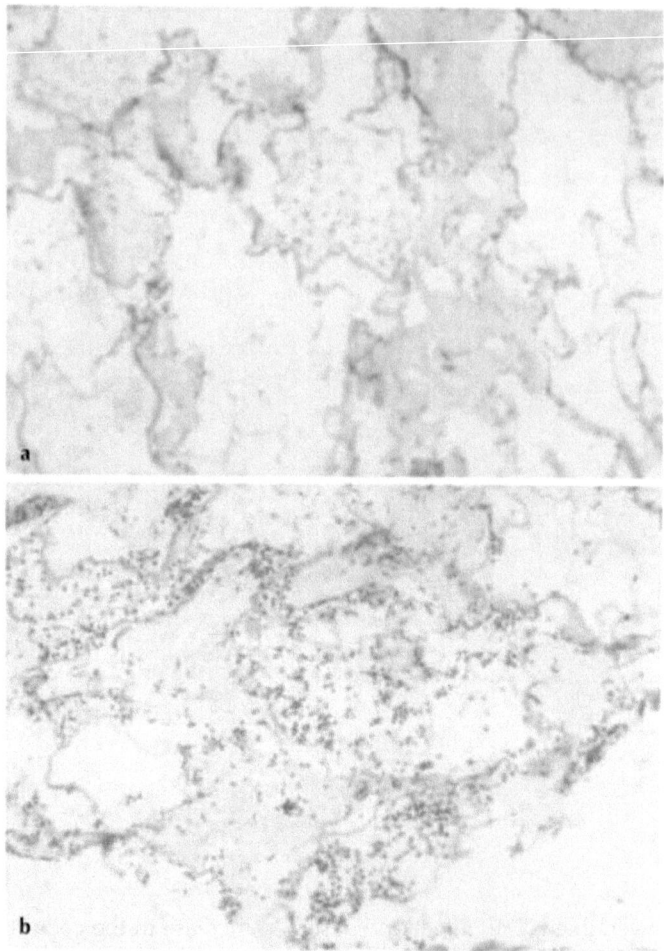

Fig. 3 a ,b. Paraffin sections of rat implanted sponges stained with hematoxylin/eosin.
a Normal saline;
b HCBP 1 mg. × 100

Discussion

Under physiological conditions, the degradation of extracellular matrix takes place during remodeling activities associated with morphogenesis and growth, as well as in particular processes like cell migration or wound healing. In these events, degradation mechanisms are balanced with matrix deposition activities, and collagenase is one of the most important enzymes involved, due to its unique ability to break down the native collagen molecule [18]. Especially in wound repair, collagenase acts not only as a débriding agent, but also as a stimulus for granulation tissue deposition and matrix remodeling [19].

Starting from these experimental findings, clinicians have used bacterial collagenase, a mixture of enzymes derived

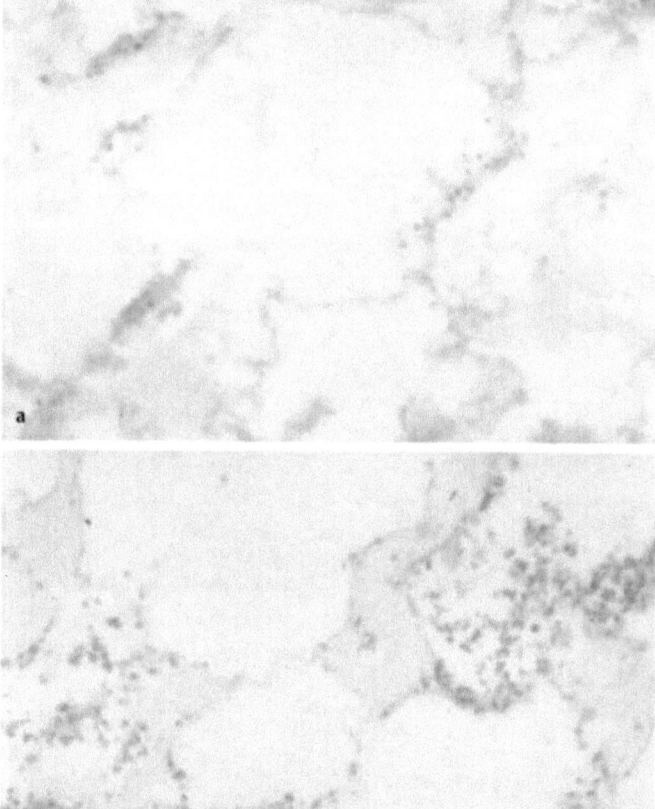

Fig. 4 a, b. Paraffin sections of rat implanted sponges stained with chloroacetate esterase. PMNs appear bright-red.
a Normal saline;
b HCBP 1 mg. × 100

mostly from *Clostridium histolyticum,* which also cleaves the native collagen molecule, as a therapeutic tool in particular pathologies, such as hyperthropic scar formation or diabetic foot ulcers [20]. The exact mechanisms by which these enzymes stimulate wound healing are partially known, and in vitro experiments have clearly demonstrated that collagen breakdown products are chemotactic for different cells involved in tissue repair [2–9,21].

In previous work [12] we demonstrated that the growth of rat fibroblasts was stimulated by HCBP in a dose-dependent manner. In this paper we confirm previous data on rat fibroblasts and report that also human fibroblasts are affected by the peptides, although a dose-dependent relationship was not clearly evident.

Fig. 5 a, b. Frozen sections of rat implanted sponges stained with diaminobenzidine. Macrophages, labeled with ED2 anti-rat antibodies and conjugated with the avidin-biotin complex, appear brown.
a HCBP 1 mg;
b HCBP 1 mg counterstained with hematoxylin. × 200

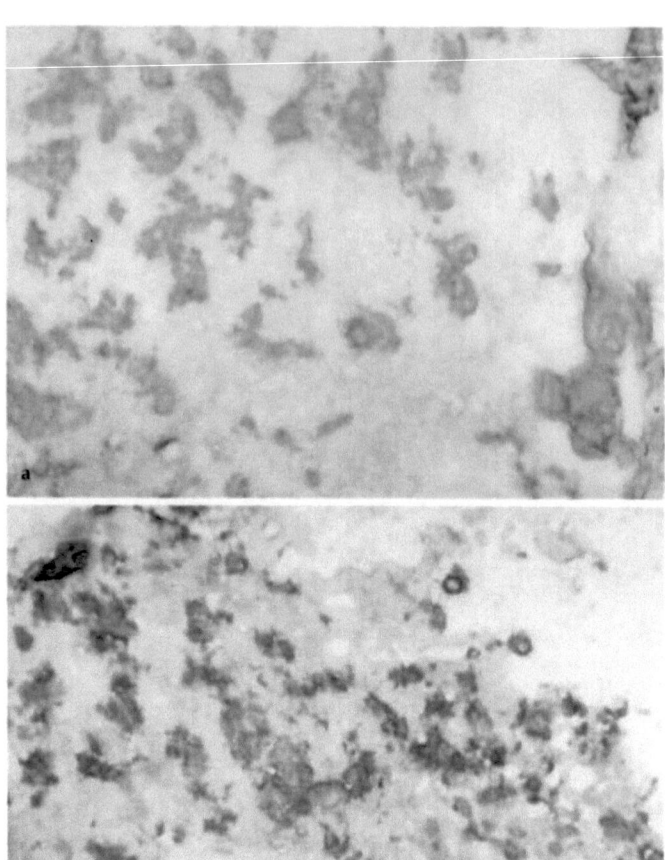

In the study conducted in vivo, we found that a single-dose administration of HCBP seemed to exert a chemotactic effect on PMNs and macrophages in a rat model of wound healing. Although we did not see an increase in collagen deposition, we believe that higher doses of the peptides and/or the use of a better, slow drug-release system may enhance the recruitment of cells other than phagocytes within the sponges, thus promoting the formation of granulation tissue and confirming the in vitro experimental findings.

In addition, it should be interesting to evaluate the collagenase and its digested product activities in an animal model of unpaired wound healing (adriamycin-treated rats). Finally, more work has to be done in order to detect the minimal amino acid sequence of collagen-derived peptides affecting the recruitment and proliferation of the different cells.

References

1. Chang C, Houck JC (1970) Demonstration of the chemotactic properties of collagen. Proc Soc Exp Biol Med 134 : 22–26
2. Postlethwaite AE, Kang AH (1976) Collagen- and collagen peptide-induced chemotaxis of human blood monocytes. J Exp Med 143 : 1299–1307
3. Postlethwaite AE, Seyer JM, Kang AH (1978) Chemotactic attraction of human fibroblasts to type I, II and III collagens and collagen-derived peptides. Proc Natl Acad Sci USA 75 : 871–875
4. Laskin DL, Kimura T, Sakakibara S, et al (1986) Chemotactic activity of collagen-like polypeptides for human peripheral blood neutrophils. J Leukoc Biol 39 : 255–266
5. Murdoch WJ, McCormick RJ (1993) Mechanisms and physiological implications of leukocyte chemoattraction into periovulatory ovine follicles. J Reprod Fertil 97 : 375–380
6. Albini A, Adelmann-Grill BC (1985) Collagenolytic cleavage products of collagen type I as chemoattractants for human dermal fibroblasts. Eur J Cell Biol 36 : 104–407
7. Laskin DL, Soltys RA, Berg RA, et al (1990) Activation of neutrophils by factors released from alveolar macrophages stimulated with collagen-like polypeptides. Am J Respir Cell Mol Biol 2 : 463–470
8. Laskin DL, Soltys RA, Berg RA, et al (1994) Activation of alveolar macrophages by native and synthetic collagen-like polypeptides. Am J Respir Cell Mol Biol 10 : 58–64
9. Wize J, Wojtecka-Lukasik E, Maslinski S (1986) Collagen-derived peptides release mast cell histamine. Agents Actions 18 : 262–265
10. Telejko E, Wrobel K, Wisniewski K, et al (1992) Pharmacological and physicochemical properties of collagen breakdown-products. Acta Neurobiol Exp 52 : 223–232
11. Woodward SC, Hermann JB (1968) Stimulation of fibroplasia in rats by bovine cartilage powder. Arch Surg 96 : 189–199
12. Cortivo R, Radice M, Brun P, et al (1995) Biological activity of human collagen breakdown products on fibroblasts. Wounds 7, (Suppl A): 38A–44A
13. Leach AA (1960) Notes on a modification of the Neuman & Logan method for the determination of the hydroxyproline. Biochem J 74 : 70–71
14. Denizot F, Lang R (1986) Rapid colorimetric assay for cell growth and survival. J Immunol Methods 89 : 271–277
15. Bradford MM (1976) A rapid and sensitive method for the quantitation of microgram quantities of protein utilizing the principle of protein-dye binding. Anal Biochem 72 : 248–254
16. Hinegardner RT (1971) An improved fluorometric assay for DNA. Anal Biochem 39 : 197–201
17. Vince DG, Hunt JA, Williams DF (1991) Quantitative assessment of the tissue response to implanted biomaterials. Biomaterials 12 : 731–736
18. Murphy G, Reynolds JJ (1993) Extracellular matrix degradation. In: Royce PM, Steinmann B (eds) Connective tissue and its heritable disorders. Wiley-Liss, New York, pp 287-316
19. Hatz RA, von Jan NCS, Schildberg FW (1994) The role of collagenase in wound healing. In: Westerhof W, Vanscheidt W (eds) Proteolytic enzymes and wound healing. Springer, Berlin Heidelberg New York, pp 75–87
20. Altman MI, Goldstein L, Horowitz S (1978) Collagenase. J Am Pediatr Assoc 68 : 11–15
21. Ranzati C, Zahn W, Thom H (1994) Bacterial collagenase and collagen breakdown products exert chemotactic effect in vitro. 4th European Tissue Repair Society Meeting, Oxford, p 77

Interview

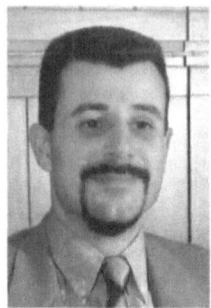

What is your hypothesis about the chemotactic effects of collagenase? Are they direct, or rather indirect due to the production of human collagen breakdown products?

Radice: Collagenase has long proven to be a valuable therapeutic tool. However, not many studies have been conducted to elucidate the mechanism(s) of action of this enzyme. It is our view that clostridial collagenase affects the wound-healing process indirectly, by means of peptides derived from the cleavage of collagen and of other ECM molecules. Actually, to investigate this point, we have planned to use eschar tissues of various origins, rather than collagen molecules, as the substrate for clostridial collagenase.

Do you think this effect is of therapeutic relevance, in addition to the wound-débriding effect of collagenase?

Radice: The in vitro findings obtained so far are very encouraging. Nevertheless, we need to run more experiments on animals in order to detect the biologically active peptide sequence(s), and to study the effect of those peptides in a model of impaired wound healing.

Human placenta has traditionally been used to heal wounds. Do your studies provide a rationale for this?

Radice: We used human placental tissue mainly because its collagen composition (types I and III) is very similar to that found in the normal skin. Otherwise, if you are using placental extracts that are not highly purified, you must consider that you do not have collagen molecules, but in fact a plethora of other substances which may show an effect in wound repair, such as growth factors or hormones.

Collagenase Therapy in the Treatment of Decubitus Ulcers

M. Nano, E. Ricci, M. De Simone, and G. Lanfranco

Summary

The authors present their experience with collagenase in the treatment of decubitus ulcers. Although they are one of the oldest known afflictions, their treatment has been of minor interest to physicians. The use of collagenase aids healing by promoting natural processes. The authors report optimal results in 900 clinical cases of decubitus ulcers among elderly patients, especially in the removal of necrotic eschar.

Introduction

Decubitus ulcers are one of the oldest known pathologies [1–3]. Among the earliest records is the Smith papyrus (3000 B.C.), in which they are accurately described, along with how they were treated with honey. In the Middle Ages, looking for an explanation of their etiology, Guglielmo da Saliceto (thirteenth century) cited immobility as the cause. In the past century, Brown-Sequard (1835) discovered that the paraplegic experimental dogs he used in his study on the effects of denervation had developed sores from remaining immobile; the reason for this he attributed to cutaneous ischemia. A century later in the United States, based on lengthy observation of his patients, Munro formed his famous "dogma" of moving the patient every 2 h, a rule that still holds today. In 1943, Mulholland was the first to realize the important role that diet – especially protein requirement – plays in the healing of wounds.

Despite their impact on social health, a specific treatment for decubitus ulcers has never come about, for two reasons. First, physicians have always been loath to deal with them. Medical history bears out this attitude in the words of the famous French physician Charcot, who, in his lectures at the Salpe-

Department of Clinical Pathophysiology and Geriatric Surgery, University of Turin, Italy

- Lesion
- Collagenase
- Lesion débrides in repair phase
- Newly formed collagen deposited (disorderly placed thin fibers mechanically inefficient)
- Collagenase
- Mature collagen (orderly placed big fibers mechanically efficient)
- Permanent scar

Table 1. Historical overview of treatment of wounds and decubitus ulcers

Author	Year	Medication
Joannes de Ketham	1491	Olive oil, honey, gum arabic, incense
Ambroise Parè	1584	Removal of necrosis, suture, medication, no boiling oil
Dominique Jean Larrey	1814	Oil, honey, sulfur and mercury salts
Astley Cooper	1825	Wine, acetic acid
James Syme	1832	Zinc sulfates, acetic acid, Mercury hydrochloride
Joseph Lister	1884	Ammonium salts, zinc, antiseptics
Alexis Carrel	1910	Sodium hypochloride
William Halstead	1917	Silver salts, mercury hydrochloride, sodium hypochloride
Hamilton Bailey	1947	Penicillin, sodium hypochloride, allantoin
George Crile, Jr.	1947	Penicillin, acetic acid

triere Hospital in Paris, expressly numbered decubitus ulcers as one of the diseases which were outside the physician's duty to treat. What is more, decubitus ulcers normally occur in elderly, debilitated, and chronically ill patients who hold only a minor interest for the physician. Second, bed sores are seen as a kind of disgraceful testimony to the nurse's poor care of her patient. This was what the equally noted Florence Nightingale meant when she spoke of decubitus as an accusation against nurses neglecting their patients. This is also why a decubitus ulcer register has never been and never will be compiled. The physician's minor interest in this pathology has been just one of the reasons why, for so many years, decubitus ulcers were treated locally with the same products used in wound care, and a specific treatment for them has never been developed.

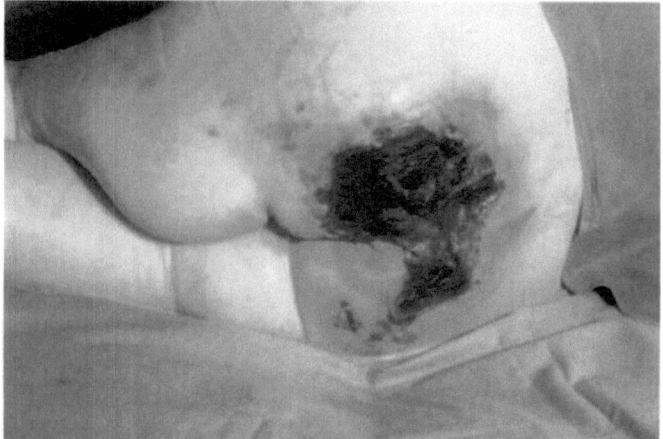

Fig. 2. Large sacral necrotic wound

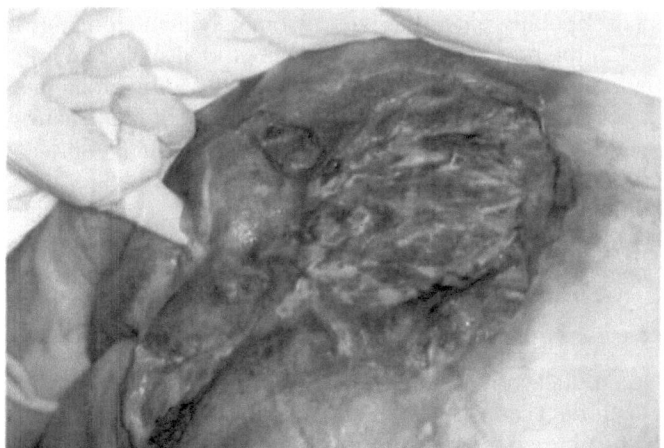

Fig. 3. Large sacral wound involving the rectum (finger inserted in the anus); débridement with collagenase

For over a decade, decubitus ulcers have represented one of the major problems in the care of elderly, bed-ridden, chronically ill, and cancer patients [4]. In hospitals for acute diseases, 3–34% of patients are affected with decubitus ulcers, while in geriatric institutes, 75% of patients present decubitus ulcers at the time of admission, especially those coming from intensive care units. In the elderly, the hospital mortality from pressure sores ranges from 23 to 57%, while the hospital mortality risk for affected patients in geriatric institutes has increased fourfold [4, 5]. This upward trend indicates the return of what had been considered a disease of the past. Another factor that has partially contributed to its rise is the progress medical science has made in keeping alive patients too fragile to support their own body weight.

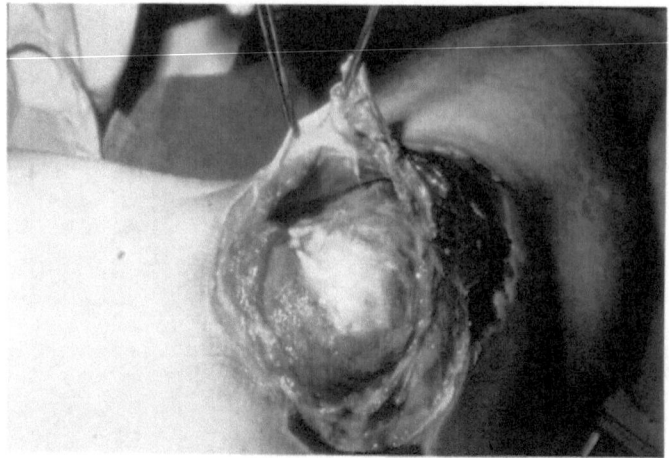

Fig. 4. Trochanteric wound with destruction of the coxofemoral joint

Going hand in hand with the scientific interest in the treatment of decubitus ulcers has been a commercial interest manifested in the production of a myriad of products all claiming to perform miracles. The consequence of this "drug proliferation", often associated with a poor knowledge of the healing processes, has been an indiscriminate use of products without a full understanding of their pharmaceutical properties or the conditions of the wound. This has led to decubitus patients being treated with an alarming number of topical drugs, in the hope that they will accomplish what the physician or the nurse has failed to. In this context we wish to underline some conclusions from our own experience:

– No product works miracles.
– No product can take the place of the nurse's preventive care or the physician's medical care.

A product is best used when the healing process is fully understood; this involves knowing what the product's properties are – how, when, and in what kind of wound it can aid healing.

In our opinion, good therapy starts with learning how to use a few currently available products very well; while we should keep an open mind about product improvements, blind belief that the newest are necessarily the best would be false. In this respect, we should recall Alessandro Manzoni's famous statement: "Not all that tomorrow brings is progress."

Débridement of Decubitus Ulcers

The healing process begins after removal of the necrotic tissue that has been inhibiting the formation of granulation tissue and cell mitosis needed for reepithelialization; devitalized tissue also forms an optimum substratum for bacterial growth [7–12]. What starts the natural process of self-débridement of a dermal wound during the initial inflammatory phases is a series of enzymes, among which is collagenase. As the natural reactions proceed, the macrophages take over the important role the neutrophils initially play. The release of chemotactic factors activates other macrophages and fibroblasts to stimulate production of collagen and neoangiogenesis. Débridement and repair thus work as two processes, so closely linked that the latter naturally takes up where the former leaves off [13]. This would justify what Sinclair and Ryan stated [14] about the fact that proteolytic enzymes are not limited to débridement alone, but also play "an intrinsic part in dermal wound repair."

Débridement with proteolytic enzymes has been widely used in the treatment of decubitus ulcers. Collagen constitutes about 75% of the dry weight of the eschar, which may be anchored to the edges and the bed of the wound by collagen strands, thereby interfering with débridement and promoting infection [4]. A small amount of collagen is digested "in loco" as part of the reactive process, but it is insufficient for self-débridement.

Many studies have tried to find products that selectively destroy necrotic tissue without, however, interfering with the granulation process or wound healing. Trypsin, chemotrypsin, streptokinase, and streptodornase all attack necrotic tissue but not native collagen [15, 16]. Collagenase has been shown to be superior to other enzymes in digesting both denatured collagen – the main component of necrotic tissue [17] – and native collagen strands that anchor residues of necrotic material to the wound bed [18]. Besides the role they play in débridement, another fundamental task of collagenase is to promote wound closure. These substances influence the balance between deposition and reabsorption of collagen in the wound and the extracellular matrix [7, 8]. Hence, by carefully controlling the synthesis and reabsorption of collagen and matrix, better repair of the wound can be achieved. Active with a pH range of 6–8, collagenase is inhibited by heavy metal ions and hexachlorophene, which should therefore not be used to disinfect the wound. Studies have not shown the formation of anti-collagenase antibodies or the event of anaphylactic reactions [4]. Collagenase has been successfully used in the treatment of many forms of skin pathologies that involve ulcers: vascular ulcers [19–22], burns in adults and children [23, 24], orthopedic pathologies and traumatology [25, 26], laser burns from cutaneous neoplastic surgical therapy [27], and radio-dermatitis [28]. Our clinical experience is based on the use of collagenase in treating decubitus ulcers with necrotic eschar.

Our Clinical Experience with Collagenase

From the vast array of treatment methods we have used in local therapy of decubitus ulcers, we have focused our attention on collagenase, because it is the product that has withstood the test of time and has proved more efficacious than many other similarly acting products that have become available in the meantime.

Our experience is based on over 900 cases of decubitus ulcers in elderly patients. In the most recent 300 cases we combined collagenase with chloramphenicol applied only in the inter-surgical phase. Débridement of necrotic ulcers, especially when large, was done in more than one session using collagenase between one treatment and the next. This eases the detachment of necrotic residue, especially of the necrotic tissues and the fibrin sticking to the periosteum at the sacrum. Application was done twice daily. In untreated cases, the interval between surgical débridement was 24 h. With the adoption of collagenase this regimen has changed. After initial cleaning, the wound was treated with the product for 4 days before being débrided again. Contrary to what used to occur, this second surgical operation has enabled us to remove all of the necrotic residue in 90% of cases. This has led to a more rapid onset of the granulation phase due to the reduction of bacterial growth, which can be seen in the reduction or remission of inflammatory signs. In no case was hypersensitivity to the product observed. In 11 cases, the patient complained of a modest burning sensation at the beginning of treatment which, however, did not lead to suspension of therapy, as has been reported in other cases by some authors [22].

In conclusion, we believe that this product represents an optimum choice in the treatment of decubitus ulcers. Nevertheless, we wish to point out that no drug can be considered a panacea in so complex and involved a treatment as that of large wounds. As our experience has shown us, an effective and widely tested drug applied correctly and appropriately helps greatly to promote a more rapid and natural healing process.

References

1. Nano M, Ricci E (1994) Le piaghe da decubito nell'anziano. Minerva Medica, Turin
2. Nano M, Ricci E, et al (1991) Le piaghe da decubito nell'anziano, sintesi di un'esperienza. Giorn Gerontol 39 : 781–788
3. Nano M, Ricci E et al (1994) Il ruolo delle collagenasi nelle piaghe da decubito. Proceedings of 8th congress of the Naz. Soc. It. Fisiop. Chirurg, pp 53–60
4. Lee LK, Ambrus JL (1975) Collagenase therapy for decubitus ulcers. Geriatrics 30 : 91–98
5. Zuccarelli GC, Berna D, et al (1990) La collagenasi nel trattamento delle ulcere da decubito nel paziente anziano ad alto rischio. Giorn Gerontol 38 : 237–241
6. Zuccarelli G, Frustaglia A, et al (1989) La collagenasi nel trattamento delle ulcere da decubito nel paziente anziano. Atti I Congr. Int. ANCAP, pp 189–191
7. Tammaro AE (1995) Il trattamento locale delle piaghe da decubito nell'anziano. Importanza della detersione e ruolo della collagenasi. Farmaci 19 : 21–26
8. Alfisi M, Boccanera D, et al. (1993) Trattamento enzimatico di ulcere di varia natura. Atti Accad Med Lombarda 39 : 1–15
9. Nano M (1988) Assistenza delle piaghe da decubito. In: Masera N, Gaggiotti G (eds) Guida all'assistenza del paziente chirurgico geriatrico. Idelson, Naples
10. Nano M, Ferrario E, et al (1989) Le piaghe da decubito nell'anziano, trattamento locale. Atti I Congr. Int. ANCAP, pp 39–52
11. Nano M, Strumia E (1982) Classificazione e trattamento delle piaghe da decubito nell'anziano. Acta Gerontol 32 : 781–788
12. Nano M, Strumia E, et al (1986) Le piaghe da decubito nell'anziano. Min Chir 41 : 1207–1210
13. Cohen IK, Diegelmann RF, et al (1992) Wound healing: biochemical and clinical aspects. Saunders, Philadelphia
14. Sinclair RD, Ryan TJ (1994) Types of chronic wound. Indications for enzymatic debridement. In: Westerhof W, Vanscheidt W (eds) Proteolytic enzymes and wound healing. Springer, Berlin Heidelberg New York, pp 7–20
15. Boxer AM, Gottesman N, et al (1969) Débridement of dermal ulcers and decubiti with collagenase. Geriatrics 24 : 75–86
16. Lazzari GB, Monteverdi AM, et al (1990) La collagenasi nel trattamento delle lesioni ulcerative torpide degli arti inferiori. Giorn Ital Dermatol Venerol 125 : 37–42
17. Helaly P, Vogt E, et al (1988) Wundheilungsstörungen und ihre enzymatische Therapie – eine Multizentrische Doppelblindstudie. Schweiz Rundschau Med (Praxis) 77 : 1428–1434
18. Varma AO, Bugatch E (1973) Débridement of dermal ulcers with collagenase. Surg Gyncecol Obstet 136 : 281–282
19. Cespa M, Donadini A, et al (1984) Una collagenasi per uso topico con medicazione semiocclusiva. Chron Dermatol 4 : 591–596
20. Pastore A, Zorzoli C (1985) Trattamento delle turbe trofiche vascolari degli arti inferiori. Min Cardioangiol 33 : 851–854
21. Brienza E, Fallacara G, et al (1990) La terapia topica delle ulcere degli arti inferiori con l'associazione collagenase-cloramfenicolo. Puglia Chir 1–6, 19–28

22. Montorio L, Vicari GB, et al (1985) Nostra esperienza sull'impiego dell'Iruxol pomata nel trattamento di ulcerazioni cutanee a varia eziologia. Giorn Ital Dermatol Venerol 120 : 29–34

23. De Luca G (1987) Uso della clostridiopeptidasi A in associazione a CAF nella terapia delle ustioni in età pediatrica. Giorn Ital Ric Clin Terapeu 8 : 64–70

24. Soroff HS, Sasvary DH (1994) Collagenase ointment and polymyxin B sulfate/Bacitracin spray versus silver sulfadiazine cream in partial thickness burns: a pilot study. J Burn Care Rehabil 15 : 13-17

25. Nepi A (1992) Il trattamento topico di lesioni cutanee con perdita di sostanza. Esperienze con una associazione di collagenasi o cloramfenicolo. Giorn Ital Ric Clin Terapeu 13 : 53–57

26. Mariotti U, Bellomo F (1984) L'associazione CAF-collagenasi-clostridiopeptidasi: suo utilizzo in ortopedia e traumatologia. Giorn Ital Ortop Traumatol 10 : 415-420

27. Tanzarella M, Calamo-Specchia R, et al (1990) Utilizzazione della collagenasi nel trattamento di lesioni conseguenti a chirurgia con LASER CO2 di neoformazioni cutanee. Folia Oncol 13 : 103–106

28. Carboni G, Longhi Gelati M, et al (1982) Esperienza clinica di un preparato topico ad attività enzimatica collagenasica nelle lesioni ulcero necrotiche cutanee. Chron Dermatol 1 : 3–17

Interview

What is the most important aspect of the preventive care of decubitus ulcers?

Nano: The most important aspect in preventing decubitus ulcers is decompression.

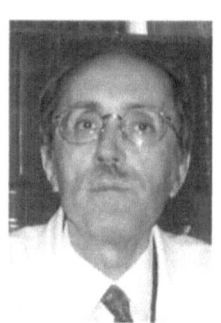

Are there any studies which make it possible to estimate the incidence and costs of decubitus ulcers in Italy?

Nano: An Italian study that reports on the incidence is that of Apostoli et al. (1988) "Observations on the epidemiology and prophylaxis of decubital lesions in reanimation." Rivista dell'Infermiere (Review of Nursing) 7 : 18–22

Can you roughly estimate the costs saved with collagenase therapy since you have fewer operations to perform?

Nano: It is difficult to calculate the costs saved with collagenases. For the phase of necrosis, the following calculations are realistic:
Time saved by nurses – 30%
Time saved by physicians – 50%
Pharmaceutical material saved – 30%

A Color CD-ROM Image Analysis System to Quantify Débridement and Healing of Ulcers

S. el Gammal[1], R. Popp[2], M. Schäfer[3], C. el Gammal[1], and P. Altmeyer[1]

Summary

The débridement activity of collagenase in decubital ulcers was evaluated in a multicenter double-blind trial according to the black-yellow-red wound classification scheme. Granulation tissue surface showed undulating curves. At first it increased due to the reduction of necrosis and fibrin/exudate, later it decreased due to epithelialization and total wound area reduction.

Introduction

In clinical trials dealing with wound healing the selection of appropriate parameters is essential. Presently, there are no internationally accepted clinical research guidelines to quantify wound healing [8].

Selection of Parameters

Various parameters have been suggested to evaluate wound quality and wound size. Measuring the maximum diameter of the wound neglects wound retraction, which occurs mainly in one direction, leading to a spindle shape of a primarily round wound during healing. Evaluating the wound area (in a picture) avoids this problem but ignores wound depth. Determination of the wound volume depends to a great extent on the positioning of the patient, especially when assessing pressure sores.

The quality of the wound surface is also of great interest. Generally, secondary healing ulcers pass through different clinical

---

[1] Department of Dermatology, Ruhr University of Bochum, Gudrunstraße 56, 44791 Bochum, Germany
[2] Clinical Research Department, Knoll AG, Ludwigshafen, Germany
[3] Technical Development Department ZET/SZ, BASF AG, Ludwigshafen, Germany

stages which each exhibit a characteristic color [9, 10]. During the late wound reaction phase black necroses can occur, which are caused by infarction after acute occlusion of arteries or arterioles. This necrotic layer often contains blood clots and sometimes is very deep, exposing large cavities with tendons and bone when removed. During the early regeneration phase yellow necroses are observed. They consist of exudate, bacteria (pus), devitalized tissue cells, collagen, and elastin. In the late regeneration phase, red vascularized granulation tissue is seen. The ulcer bed is now clean and the wound space is filled by cellular elements and newly formed collagen and ground substance. Finally, pale, pinky epithelialization progresses from the wound borders and a scar is formed. Several recent studies [1, 18, 19] have used a colorimetric "black-yellow-red (BYR)" classification scheme, which focuses on the wound surface, excluding epithelialization for practical reasons. A gradual shift of the ulcer surface from black, solid necrotic areas to fibrinoid/necrotic regions, which are yellow, and finally to healthy red granulation tissue is assumed.

Patient Follow-up

Heterogeneity of wounds and treatment regimens, a variety of underlying diseases, and poor patient compliance complicate the collection of reproducible and comparable data about wound healing. Epidemiological data on patients with chronic ulcers illustrate these problems. In a community survey of 477 patients with venous leg ulcers, the duration of the ulcer ranged from 1 week to 63 years, and its size from 0.1 to 117 cm^2 [12]. Healing time varied considerably, and recurrence rates were very high. In another epidemiological study, in 49% of patients re-ulceration occurred within 3 months after hospital discharge [13]. Ulcer size, duration of an ulceration, the patient's age, and deep vein involvement are major prognostic factors for the healing time in venous leg ulcers [17].

In patients with pressure sores the healing period can last for about 1 year [20]. This long healing time is a major problem in wound healing trials, as many patients die during follow-up or are referred to other units or nursing homes. According to our experience, even trials with a short observation period are difficult to manage as the course of the disease varies considerably and requires different treatment regimes.

Quantification of Wound Healing

In the past years, various approaches to documenting and quantifying wound healing have been used (Table 1).

Table 1. Proposed parameters for wound healing

Proposed method	Disadvantages	Information provided
Clinical assessment	Subjective	Qualitative and quantitative
Foil planimetry	Patient discomfort wound contamination	Only quantitative (2-D)
Casting	Accuracy Wound secrete interaction	Only quantitative (3-D)
Photography	Geometric perspective distortion Unequal illumination	Qualitative and quantitative
Video image analysis	Limited resolution	Qualitative and quantitative (2-D)
Stereophoto-grammetry	Complex precision equipment	Qualitative and quantitative (3-D)

Clinical assessment of wound healing at fixed intervals is the simplest and most widely performed evaluation procedure. The wound surface, its size, shape, and borders have been used as parameters. The subjectivity and wide interobserver variability are great disadvantages of this approach.

Planimetry requires thorough delineation of the wound edge on a transparent sheet placed on the wound surface. Later, series of sheets may be superimposed to objectively assess the healing process. When the delineated sheets are cut out, planimetric evaluation is possible using gravimetry. Although foil-planimetry may seem acceptable, it causes discomfort to the patient and increases the risk of wound contamination. The main disadvantage of this method is that it focuses solely on quantitative evaluation of the total wound surface and disregards wound surface quality.

Casting methods are useful for wound volume evaluation. Silicon replicas [16, 22] or dental impression materials [3] have been the most commonly used. The wound volume can be measured by immersing the cast (Archimedes' principle). Surface topography can be quantified using profilometry [15, 22]. Unfortunately, accurate casts of superficial wounds on convex or concave surfaces are difficult to obtain, and the interaction of the cast with the wound secretion presents unsolved problems.

Photography avoids contact with the lesion and thereby prevents contamination and tissue damage. It can be performed

quickly at different time points and stages of healing and without inconvenience for the patient. Several investigators can judge the pictures independently of each other, providing a better reproducibility and objectivity.

Furthermore, photographs are well suited to evaluate both qualitative and quantitative aspects of the wound surface. For this purpose, lighting conditions must be kept constant in follow-up pictures.

Polaroid systems have the advantage of instant prints and therefore provide significantly fewer logistical problems with respect to processing, storing, and identification of the photographs in a multicenter setting. Their greatest disadvantage is the poor resolution and a low depth of field in comparison to 35-mm slides taken with a closed aperture. In our experience, this is also true for specially designed camera systems like the Acmel® camera [6] or the Medical Nikkor® 35-mm camera.

Morphometric evaluation has to struggle with the geometrical perspective distortion on photographs. This optic geometrical error can be corrected in flat wounds by using transparent graph paper or a reference scale. Palmer et al. [14] have shown that assessment of an irregular shape on a plane model is quite reliable as long as the camera is within 10° of the right angle to the object.

In recent years, **computer image analysis** has gained new application fields in medicine. Computerized wound analysis has been propagated by Eriksson et al. [7]. Bengtsson et al. [1] have shown that computerized wound analysis reduces both intra- and interobserver variability and is reliable in comparison to clinical assessment. In an ideal situation, wounds of approximately the same size are studied by the image analysis system.

Most CWA systems consist of a video camera, a frame grabber, a computer, and an image analysis software [11, 14]. The resolution of standard video technology is quite low and varies between 512 × 512 and 1024 × 768 pixels per image. A fixed camera-to-wound distance can lead to resolution problems when the size of the wounds varies considerably. If the preadjusted image area was 20×20 cm^2, a small wound of 1×1 cm^2 would represent only 0.25% of the total image surface. If the image area had 262 000 pixels, the region of interest would have 655 pixels. This leads to significant limitations, especially in a multicenter setting.

Additional volumetric information on convex and concave surfaces can be gained by **stereophotogrammetry** [2, 7] when pairs of stereo photos of a wound are available. Using two fix-mounted cameras, stereo pictures can be photographed simultaneously. Alternatively, the pictures are photographed sequentially, using a single camera on an optical bench. The distance between both images is used for further calculations. In a first step prominent points have to be recognized in both stereo pictures. The parallactic displacement of a homologous point in both pictures is then used to calculate its depth. To avoid systematic errors during depth measurements, high-quality optic camera lenses without astigmatism are necessary. Furthermore, sophisticated mechanical precision equipment or complex time-consuming computer evaluations are needed to correlate both stereo pictures and evaluate the parallactic displacement for every point within the picture. At present, these problems are serious limitations to this method.

A New CD-ROM Color Wound Analysis System (CD-CWA) Suitable for Multicenter Trials

Wound analysis should assess the wound surface quality and wound size simultaneously. We designed a color wound analysis system which uses high-resolution images for precise wound quantification. This system has been validated and is presently being used in several multicenter studies. These studies focus on the evaluation of the wound débridement, since pharmacologically induced acceleration of débridement has been demonstrated to decrease healing time significantly [21, 23].

Photographic Documentation

Photographic films with fine granularity are particularly suitable for documenting wounds of greatly varying sizes because this analogue medium has a high detail resolution. We used 35-mm slides because they provide an excellent resolution.

Our camera system consists of a Canon 35-mm body (EOS100®), an ML 3 ring flash, and a 50-mm macro lens. This camera is suitable for photographic documentation in a multicenter setting. To limit the length of the photo session, the camera is equipped with an automatic film drive. Misfunction is minimized by an automatic adjustment to film sensitivity and shutter blockage when the film is not inserted correctly, already exposed, or rewound. A camera back was used, which fades in the date for identification of the photographs.

Fig. 1. Every color pixel in an image is a combination of red, green, and blue intensities (RGB). Alternatively, the color can be described by an HSI color representation system. *H,* Hue; *S,* color saturation; *I,* whiteness intensity

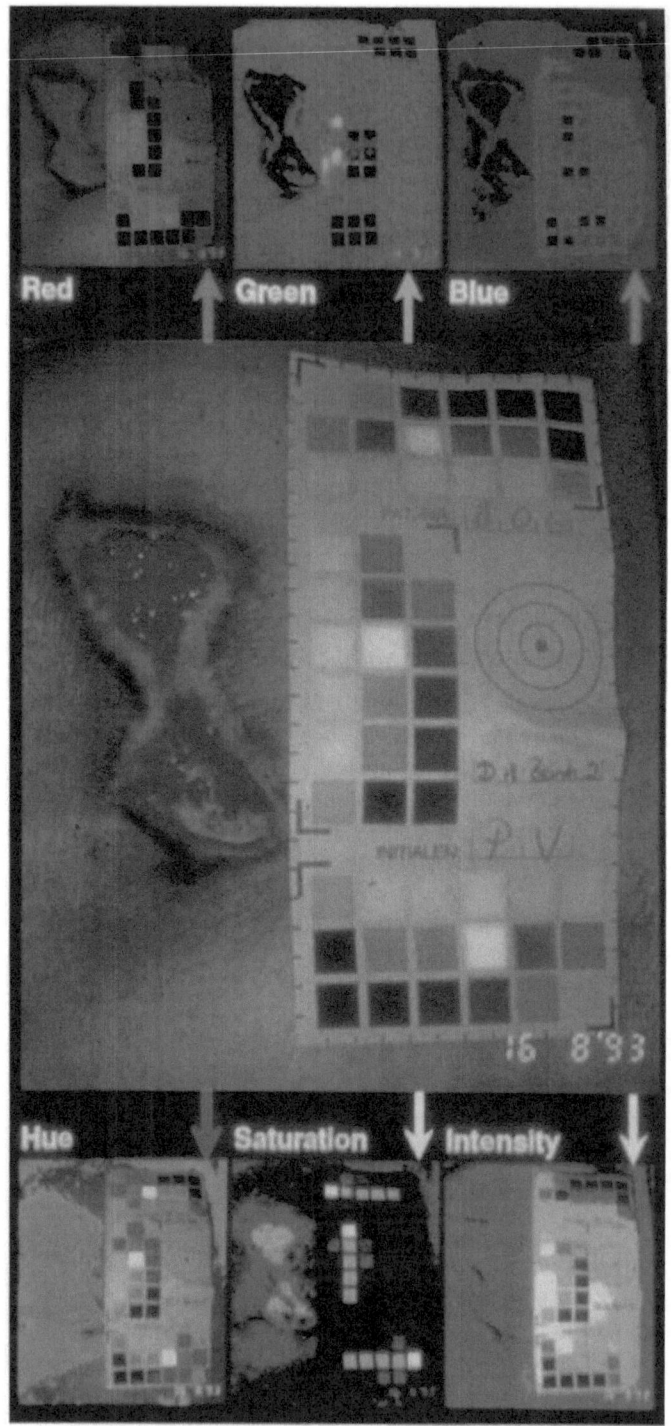

We chose a distance of 40 cm for all photographs by fixing the distance ring. The infrared distance meter emits an acoustic signal when this distance is met. A fixed aperture of 16, a shutter speed of 1/125 s, and an automatic TTL flash exposure is used. We suggest using 35-mm slides, because film development is standardized. A medium film sensitivity (21 DIN) was selected in order to assure rapid recharging of the flash. In comparison to other cameras and video systems, this camera set-up is easy to use in a multicenter setting and provides pictures with a good depth of field (aperture of 16 and TTL control of the flash).

The position of the patient and the investigator are recorded at baseline. This position should be reproduced as exactly as possible during all follow-up visits. The reference scale is fixed to the skin at the border of the lesion vertically (as seen by the investigator). The infrared distance meter is activated by gently pressing the shutter. When the camera is moved up and down along the vertical axis of the wound surface, an acoustic signal is heared as soon as the selected 40 cm distance is reached.

Reference Scale

We developed a reference scale to calibrate distances and to compensate for color variation due to exposure and/or film emulsion in each image [5]. The patient number and initials can also be documented on this self-adhesive paper card (see Fig. 1). Concentric circles with 8, 16, and 24 mm diameters are used for distance calibration. If these circles turn out to be elliptic on the photographs, there is significant distortion and perspective error in the images. Identical reference color blocks are included on the reference card at three different positions. This redundance ensures that a complete set of all colors can be used for reference, regardless of the perspective.

Multicenter Monitoring

All centers were thoroughly instructed on how to handle the camera and to take the pictures in a reproducible and standardized manner. Throughout the trial there was continuous control of correct function of the camera, and detailed advice on how to achieve optimal pictures was provided. Intense monitoring is an essential prerequisite and can reduce missing data due to logistic and quality-related problems of the applied technique and the quality of the pictures.

Processing of the Films and CD-ROM Transfer

All exposed films were sent to the same processing laboratory. The best 24- × 36-mm slides were then selected from each photo session and matched. The following criteria must be met:

1. Identification must be unambiguous, based on the reference scale and patient number, study code, and patient initials.
2. The photo is taken at 40 cm distance (1:6 scale) with sufficient lighting.
3. The entire wound surface is seen.
4. At least one color reference block is in the vicinity of the wound.

The selected slides were digitized on "write-once" Kodak photo compact discs (CD). Every picture is accessible in five different resolutions (192 × 128 to 3072 × 2048 pixels with 16 million colors). At high resolution, the size of a single image file ranges up to 6 MBytes.

Color Analysis

In most computer applications, pictures are treated as two-dimensional arrays of pixels. In black-and-white pictures every pixel is visualized as a gray spot. Its gray level is represented in the array as an integer number between black (i.e., "0") and white (i.e., "255"). To improve the differentiation of small gray-level differences for the eye, some applications map every gray level to a specific color [4].

In true color images, every pixel has a separate red, green, and blue intensity level (Fig. 2). This RGB color coding is quite abstract and does not correspond to the categories of human color perception [5]. We prefer to use the HSI (hue, saturation, intensity) color coding system, because it is more intuitive than the RGB system (Fig. 1). The hue describes the basic color on a color circle of 360°, analogous to a clock face. Red corresponds to 0°, yellow to 60°, green to 120°, azure to 180°, blue to 240°, and violet to 300°. The saturation describes the color density, whereas the intensity refers to the amount of whiteness in the color. All available colors are included in a three-dimensional ovaloid (Fig. 2), where Hue and Saturation are polar coordinates and the Intensity is orthogonally oriented.

Each of the three wound surface qualities (black necrosis; yellow, fibrinoid/necrotic area; and clean red granulation tissue) can be described by a characteristic three-dimensional region in the three-dimensional HSI ovaloid. The granulation tissue typically fills the compact "red" region and is surrounded by a shell-shaped fibrinoid/necrotic region. The region of black necrotic tissue exhibits low intensity values. Poorly illuminated granulation tissue therefore is at risk of being assessed as necrosis.

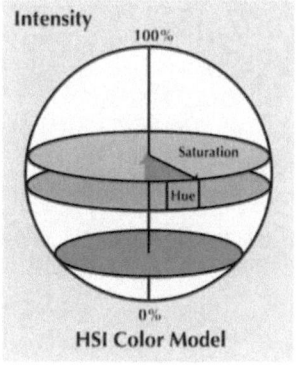

Fig. 2. The HSI color representation system forms a 3-D ovaloid, where all possible colors are included. *H*, Hue; *S*, color saturation; *I*, whiteness intensity. By moving in a radial direction the saturation of the color changes, by moving circularly its hue changes. The whiteness intensity is vertically oriented in the color ovaloid

Since these defined HSI color regions remain constant for the assessment of all wound photos, a constant and homogeneous illumination is necessary to achieve high reliability in wound area classification.

Wound Evaluation Steps

We use a commercially available image analysis software (e.g., AnalySIS, Soft-Imaging Software GmbH, Münster, FRG, or ConceptVI, Graftek, Le Moulin de l'Image, Mirmande, France) which supports virtual image buffers of different size, image filtering, and other standard procedures. The image analysis protocol was built by combining different library functions.

Images are loaded from the photo-CD, and the wound area (region of interest) is cut out interactively. On every image the reference card is used to correct for geometry, film emulsion, and exposure in the region of interest. The mean intensity (I) of the picture is calculated and corrected to a standard intensity of 128. The ulcer outline is then determined interactively. The ulcer area is classified pixel-wise into black necrosis, fibrinoid/necrotic wound area, and clean red granulation tissue. When the pictures are well illuminated and exhibit few reflexes, 60–90% (mean 80%) of the ulcer surface can be correctly classified. By cyclic region growing of the directly detected granulation tissue, fibrinoid, and black necrosis, all unclassified areas become classified.

Figure 3 shows a pressure sore in the gluteal region at baseline. The detected classified regions are marked on the inserts. Granulation tissue is represented as red area, black necrosis as blue area, and the fibrin-covered or yellow necrotic wound surface as yellow area. Figures 5 and 6 show the same pressure sore at baseline and after 4, 8, 11, 17, and 22 days. Correspondingly, black necrosis, fibrinoid/necrotic regions, and

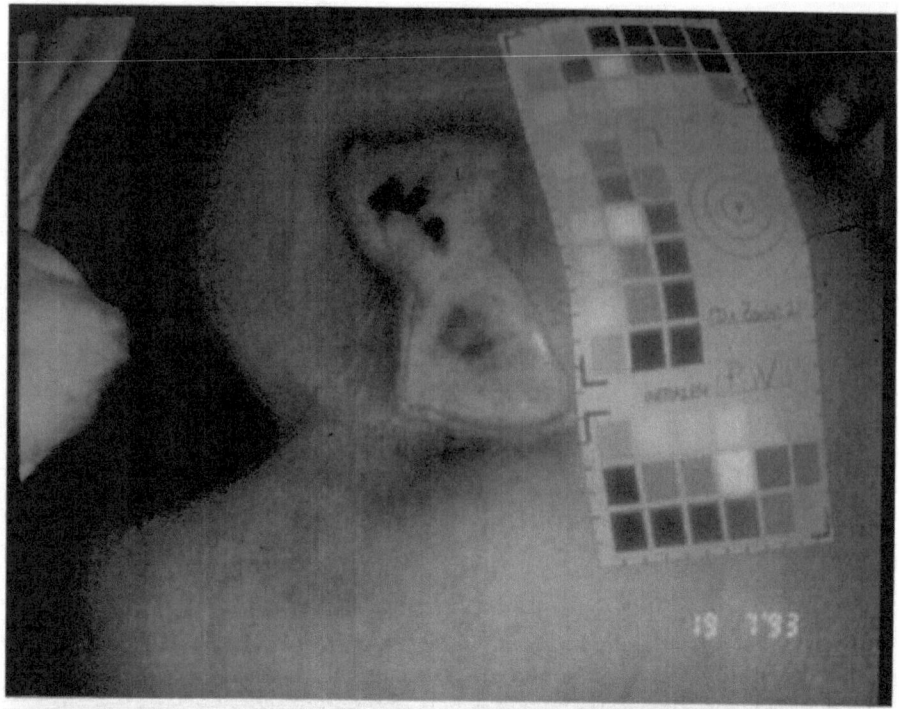

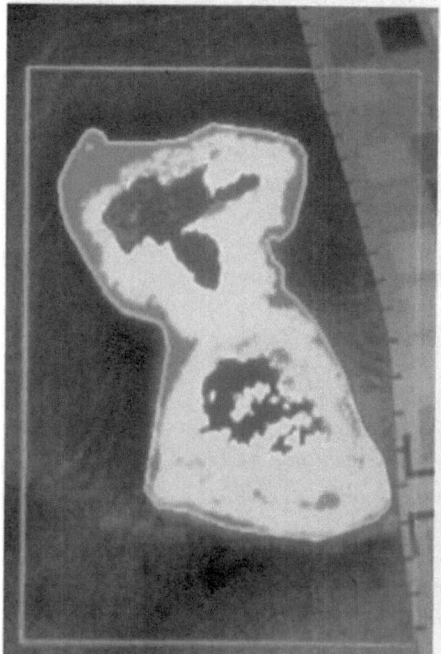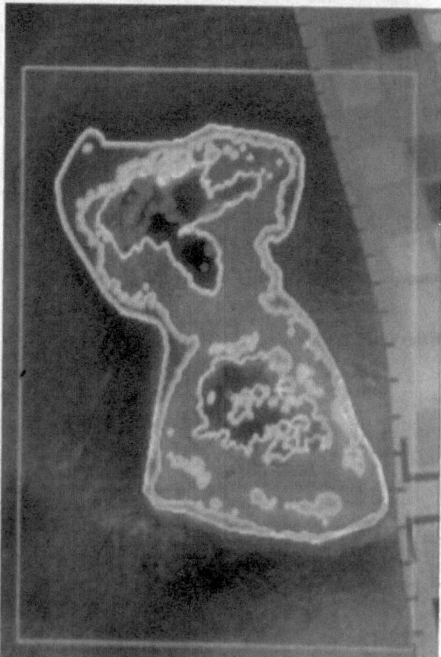

Fig. 3. Decubital sore at baseline. Original image *(top)*. The CD-CWA program has detected granulation tissue *(red)*, necrosis *(blue)*, and fibrinoid exudate *(yellow)*. In the *inserts,* these surfaces are filled *(left)* and outlined *(right)*

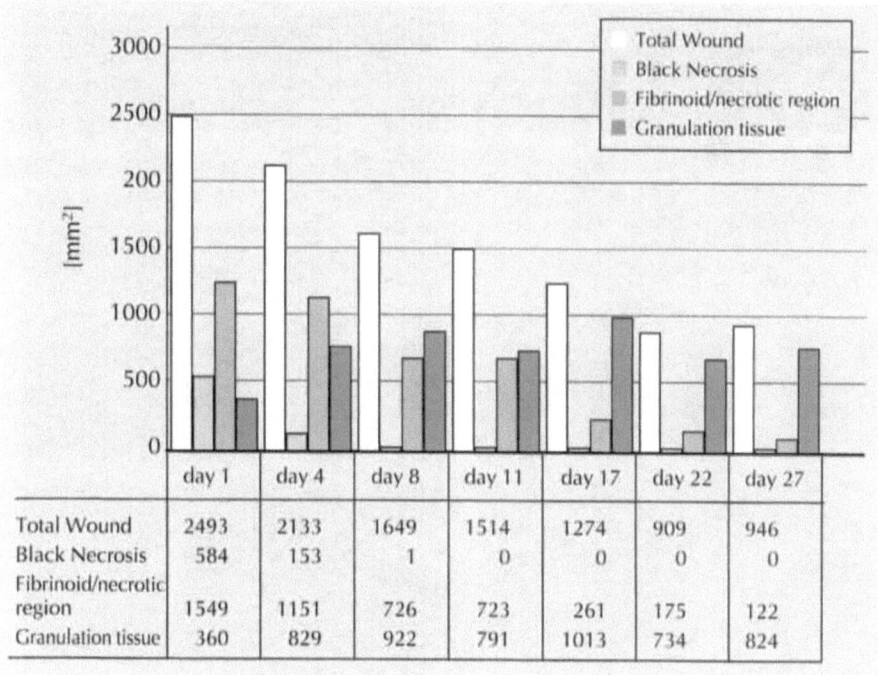

	day 1	day 4	day 8	day 11	day 17	day 22	day 27
Total Wound	2493	2133	1649	1514	1274	909	946
Black Necrosis	584	153	1	0	0	0	0
Fibrinoid/necrotic region	1549	1151	726	723	261	175	122
Granulation tissue	360	829	922	791	1013	734	824

granulation tissue have been marked on Fig. 6. Figure 4 shows follow-up area measurements of a single gluteal decubital ulcer. Within 26 days, the total wound surface has decreased significantly by retraction and epithelialization from the borders. Black necrosis and the fibrinoid/necrotic surface decreased during this time period. We found that the granulation tissue surface shows particularly interesting undulating curves. We believe that this is due to two concurring effects: the area of granulation increases at first mainly due to the reduction of black necrosis and fibrinoid/necrotic regions, while later on it decreases due to epithelialization and total wound area reduction.

Fig. 4. Absolute area *(mm²)* of the total wound surface, granulation tissue, necrosis, and fibrinoid exudate at baseline *(day 1)*, day 4, day 8, day 11, day 17, and day 22. Note that the necrotic area decreases rapidly. The granulation tissue area exhibits an undulating curve

Evaluation of Leg Ulcers

Evaluation of leg ulcers is more complicated than that of gluteal pressure sores because of the curvature of the lower leg. The geometric perspective distortion and the intensity decline due to the curvature of the leg can be corrected by the image analysis software as follows: the convexity of the region of interest (e.g., the leg) is approximated by a corresponding geometrical body (e.g., a cylinder). A least-square fit illumination correction over the picture enhances significantly the classification into HSI color regions.

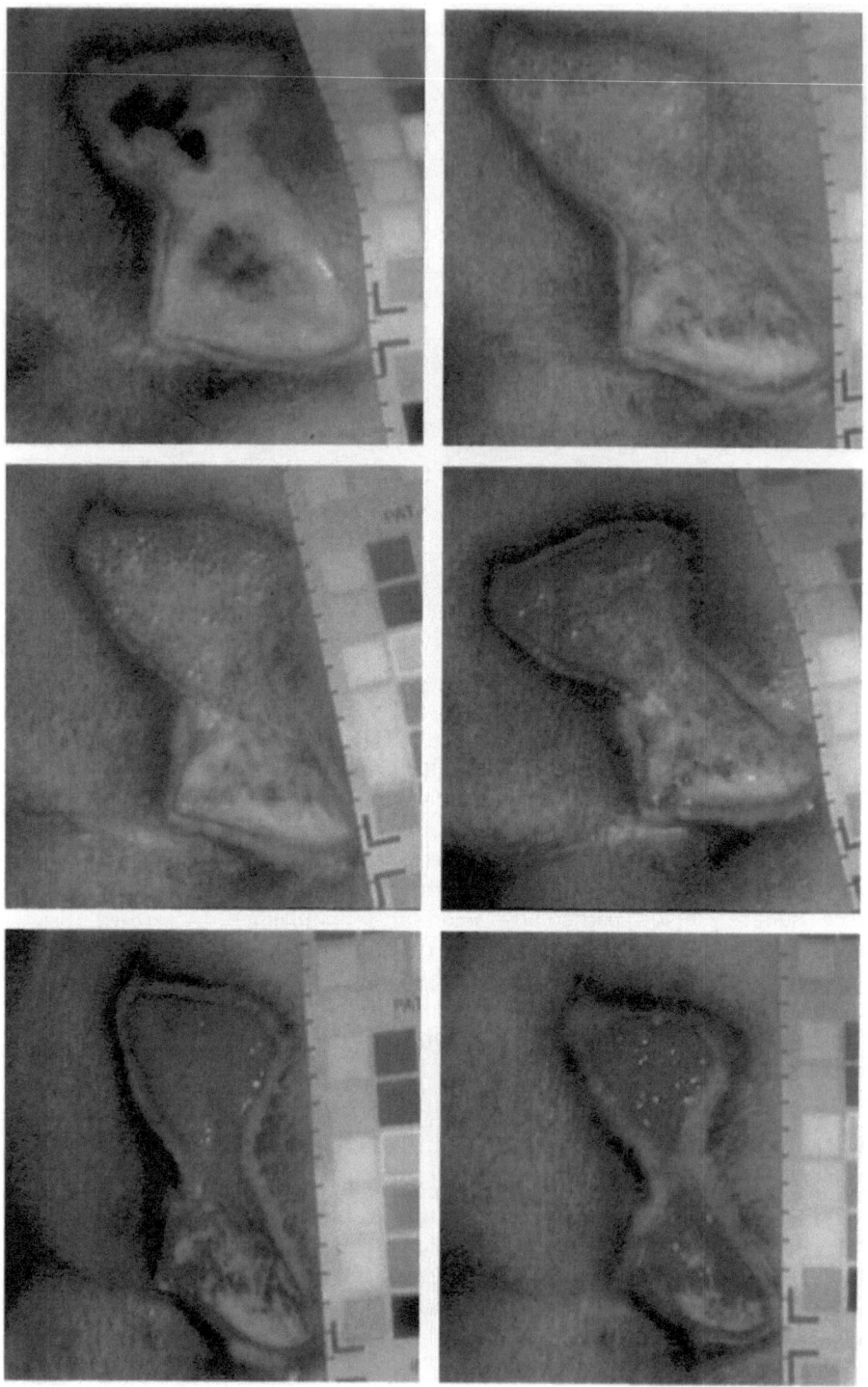

Fig. 5. Decubital sore on CD-ROM pictures at baseline *(top left)*, day 4 *(top right)*, day 8 *(middle left)*, day 11 *(middle right)*, day 17 *(bottom left)*, and day 22 *(bottom right)*. Note the ulcer débridement

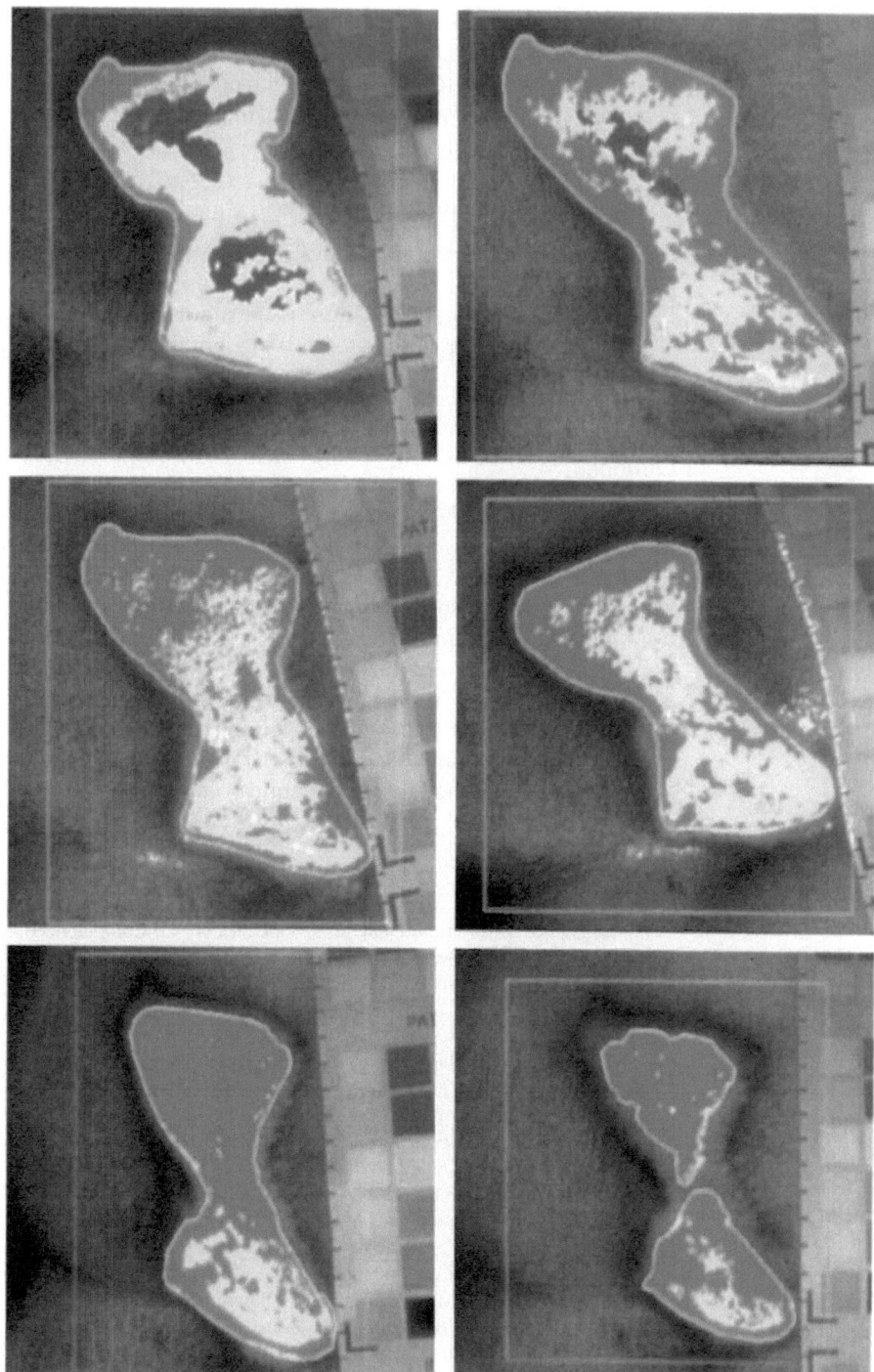

Fig. 6. Decubital sore at baseline *(top left)*, day 4 *(top right)*, day 8 *(middle left)*, day 11 *(middle right)*, day 17 *(bottom left)*, and day 22 *(bottom right)*. The CD-CWA program has detected granulation tissue *(red)*, necrosis *(blue)*, and fibrinoid exudate *(yellow)*

The ulcer can be delimited interactively and the evaluation procedures described above are applied. Finally, the detected regions are decomposed into lines which are multiplied by the geometric correction factor (due to the cylindric approximation).

Limitations in Wound Image Analysis

Classification of the wound surface into the mentioned categories can, however, create problems, for example, when thin blood crusts overlying granulation tissue simulate necrosis or when hyperergic vasculitis, resembling granulation tissue, imitates necrosis [5].

Outlook

We believe that CD-ROM color wound analysis is a good tool for objective assessment of wound healing of ulcers. The method is well suited for widespread use in clinical practice. More experience with this kind of standardized documentation and evaluation provides a basis for the development of new techniques. By optimizing the quality of photographic images the accuracy of CD-CWA can be further improved. We think that in the future, the development of stereo CD-ROM color wound analysis could integrate the evaluation of wound quality, wound area, and wound volume.

References

1. Bengtsson E, Engström N, Hellgren L, Vincent J (1995) Computerized wound analysis – a new method for assessment of healing. In: Altmeyer P, Hoffmann K, el Gammal S, Hutchinson J (eds) Wound healing and skin physiology. Springer, Berlin Heidelberg New York, pp 481–483
2. Bulstrode CJK, Goode AW, Scott PJ (1986) Stereophotogrammetry for measuring rates of cutaneous healing: a comparison with conventional techniques. Clin Sci 71 : 437-443
3. Covington JS, Griffin JW, Mendius RK, et al (1989) Measurement of pressure ulcer volume using dental impression materials: suggestion from the field. Phys Ther 69 : 690–694
4. el Gammal S, Hoffmann K, Höss A, Hammentgen R, Altmeyer P, Ermert H (1992) New concepts and developments in high-resolution ultrasound. In: Altmeyer P, el Gammal S, Hoffmann K (eds) Ultrasound in dermatology. Springer, Berlin Heidelberg New York, pp 399–442
5. el Gammal S, Brand M, el Gammal C, Hoffmann K, Altmeyer P (1995) A color image analysis system (CD-CWA) for the quantification of wound healing in multicenter trials. In: Altmeyer P, Hoffmann K, el Gammal S, Hutchinson J (eds) Wound healing and skin physiology. Springer, Berlin Heidelberg New York, pp 485–496
6. Engström N, Hansson F, Hellgren L, Jahansson T, Nordin B, Vincent J, Wahlberg A (1990) Computerized image analysis. In: Wadström T, Eli-

asson I, Holder I, Ljung A (eds) Pathogenesis of wound and biomaterial-associated infections. Springer, Berlin Heidelberg New York, pp 189–192

7. Eriksson G, Eklund AE, Torlegård K, Dauphin E (1979) Evaluation of leg ulcer treatment with stereophotogrammetry. Br J Dermatol 101 : 123–131

8. ETRS Working Parties Consensus Paper on Wound Healing Studies (1993) Unpublished data, distributed during the Joint Meeting of the European and American Tissue Repair Society, Amsterdam, August 22–25

9. Hellgren L, Vincent J (1986) A classification of dressing and preparations for the treatment of wounds by second intention based on stages in the healing process. Care Sci Pract 4 : 13–17

10. Hellgren L, Vincent J (1993) Débridement – an essential step in wound-healing. In: Westerhof W (ed) Leg ulcers: diagnosis and treatment. Elsevier Science, Amsterdam, pp 305–312

11. Mekkes JR, Westerhof W, Van Riet Paap E, Estevez O (1993) A new computer images analysis system designed for evaluating wound débriding products. In: Proc of the 2nd Europ Conf on Advances in Wound Management. Macmillan Magazines, Harrogate

12. Moffatt C, Franks PJ, Oldroyd M, Bosanquet N, Brown P, Greenhalgh RM, McCollum CN (1992) Community clinics for leg ulcers and impact on healing. Br Med J 305 : 1389–1392

13. Monk BE, Sarkany I (1982) Outcome of treatment of venous stasis ulcers. Clin Exp Dermatol 7 : 397–400

14. Palmer RM et al (1989) A digital video technique for radiographs and monitoring ulcers. J Photogr Sci 37 : 75–79

15. Plassmann P, Jojnes BF (1992) Measuring leg ulcers by colour-coded structured light. J Wound Care 3 : 35–38

16. Pories WJ, Schear EW, Jordan DR, Chase J, Parkinson G, Whittaker R, Strain WH, Rob C (1966) The measurement of human wound healing. Surgery 59 : 821–824

17. Skene AI, Smith JM, Dore CJ, Charlett A, Lewis JD (1992) Venous leg ulcers: a prognostic index to predict time to healing. Br Med J 305 : 1119–1121

18. Stotts NA (1990) Seeing red and yellow and black. The three-color concept of wound care. Nursing 20 : 59–61

19. Thomas S (1990) Wound management and dressings. Pharmaceutical Press, London

20. Westerhof W, van Ginkel CJW, Cohen EB, Mekkes JR (1990) Prospective randomized study comparing the débriding effect of krill enzymes and a non-enzymatic treatment in venous leg ulcers. Dermatologica 181 : 293–297

21. Yamashita S, Ohmi A, Harnada Y, et al (1989) Effects of ointment containing collagenase derived from *Achromobacter isophagus* (ACR-59 ointment) upon burn, decubital ulcer, open and cut wound studied with experimental rat models. Pharmacometrics 37 : 313–327

22. Zahouani H, Assoul M, Janod P, Mignot J (1992) Theoretical and experimental study of wound healing: application to leg ulcers. Med Biol Eng Comput 30 : 234–239

23. Zimmermann WE (1972) The importance of collagenase for the local treatment of major burns. In: Mandel I (ed) Collagenase. Gordon and Breach Science, London, pp 131ff

Interview

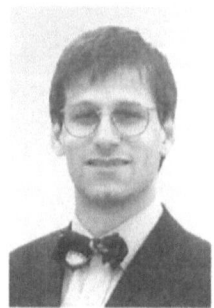

What are the most important results of your study?

el Gammal: We have developed a new method for studying ulcer débridement, based on evaluation of both wound area and wound quality. Using image analysis of CD-ROM pictures, we can quantify different parameters of healing: wound size, area of granulation tissue, area of fibrinoid/necrotic tissue, and area of black necrosis.

What are the main advantages of color image analysis using compact-disk technology (CD-ROM) for the evaluation of wound healing?

el Gammal: Using high-resolution digitization of photographic slides on CD-ROM, we can overcome the problem of poor resolution in the digitized picture when the ulcers are small.

Why didn't you zoom in on the ulcers?

el Gammal: This study was done in a multicenter environment. We therefore had to keep things simple and used a fixed photographic setting (40 cm wound-camera distance) independent of the size of the ulcer. Furthermore, the fixed 40 cm distance keeps perspective distortion low.

Congratulations on your excellent sharp pictures. How did you overcome the problem of blurred pictures, particularly in ulcers on the curved lower leg?

el Gammal: We selected our fixed camera setting in such a way that we obtained a great depth of field (flash illumination, aperture of 16, 1/125 s exposure time).

Do you see future noninvasive technical developments which will allow you to evaluate not only changes of the wound surface but also of the wound depth?

el Gammal: Interferometry is a promising method for evaluating wound volume noninvasively. I believe, however, that stereo CD-ROM color wound analysis could integrate the evaluation of wound quality, wound area, and wound volume in the near future.

Quantitative and Objective Evaluation of Wound Débriding Properties of Collagenase in a Necrotic Ulcer Animal Model

J. R. Mekkes, J. E. Zeegelaar, and W. Westerhof

Summary

The wound cleansing properties of collagenase in several new galenic formulations were compared to another commercially available enzymatic débriding agent in an observer-blind, placebo-controlled animal study using a necrotic ulcer pig model. Collagenase was significantly better in removing necrosis than placebo control ointment.

Introduction

The number of wound care materials available on the market is growing rapidly. Making a choice can be difficult. To provide clinicians with the evidence that can guide them in their choice, randomized controlled clinical trials are needed. The same type of studies are necessary in the development phase of new products.

In general, when it is technically feasible, we prefer to test new products in an animal model first, because it is difficult to investigate wound healing products in human subjects, for several reasons. The first reason is the extreme variability in wounds and patients. There are a lot of confounding factors that can influence the outcome of a clinical trial, such as wound size, depth, localization, vascularisation, duration, cause, previous treatments, the patients general health, nutritional state, use of other medication, etc. Because of this variability, large numbers of patients per treatment group have to be included. The exclusion criteria should be strict to avoid these confounding factors, which makes it difficult to find patients. Usually these trials are very time-consuming, and expensive.

A second problem is the lack of objective evaluation methods. The evaluation method should be appropriate for the

Department of Dermatology, Academisch Medisch Centrum, Meibergdreef 9, 1105 AZ Amsterdam

wound type and the wound healing phase (débridement phase, granulation tissue formation, epithelialization phase, or remodeling phase) [1]. If a product is designed for use in the epithelialization phase, than the time required for complete wound healing, or the reduction in wound size within a certain time limit, can be used as a primary outcome parameter. If a product is designed for wound cleaning, the wound size is an useless parameter, because wound size can remain exactly the same or increase slightly during the débridement phase, while important qualitative changes occur: the yellow or greenish black layers of necrotic epidermal and dermal structures, consisting of collagen and other extracellular matrix proteins and fibrin are removed and gradually replaced by healthy red granulation tissue [2]. To solve this problem, we developed a digital image analysis technique to measure the shift from black/yellow necrosis to red granulation tissue objectively [3–9]. The combination of this evaluation technique with an animal wound model makes it possible to investigate wound care products designed for wound cleaning in an objective way, within a short time period. The pig is the most appropriate animal because the structure of pig skin resembles human skin more than any other laboratory animal [10]. And because of the large test area, more than one product can be tested simultaneously in the same model.

This chapter describes how the animal model can be used to study new galenic formulations of collagenase, in a placebo-controlled, observer-blind way. Since these studies are still ongoing, we focused more on describing the model than on the preliminary results.

Methods

Animal Model

Ten female Dutch N.Y. pigs weighing 25 kg were used. On arrival the pigs were washed and placed in quarantine for 7 days during which each animal was submitted to a daily health inspection. In this period the animals could adjust to the new environment. Under total anesthesia in each swine 5 x 5 cm wounds were made on the back, with a Brown electrical dermatome. Before wounding the hairs were clipped. Immediately before operation the pigs were anesthetized with isoflurane, oxygen, and nitrous oxide via a face mask, intubated, and then maintained on close circuit anesthesia using a mixture of oxygen, nitrous oxide and isoflurane. During the operation, all vital functions were monitored. The animals received Ringer's glucose solution and adequate anesthetics (0.005 mg/kg su-

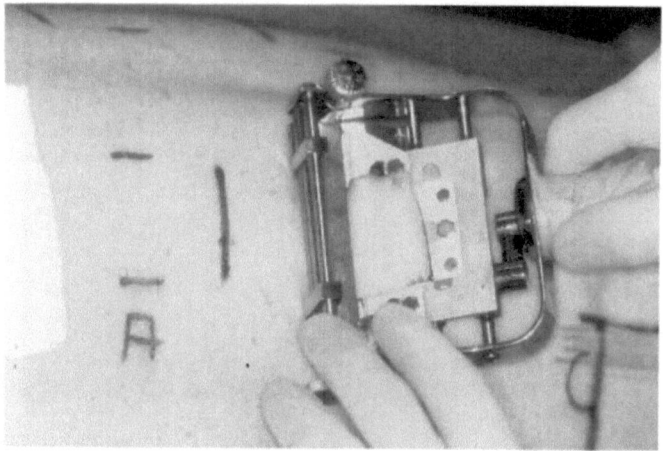

Fig. 1. Excision of 2.5 mm of the skin, using a Brown electrical dermatome

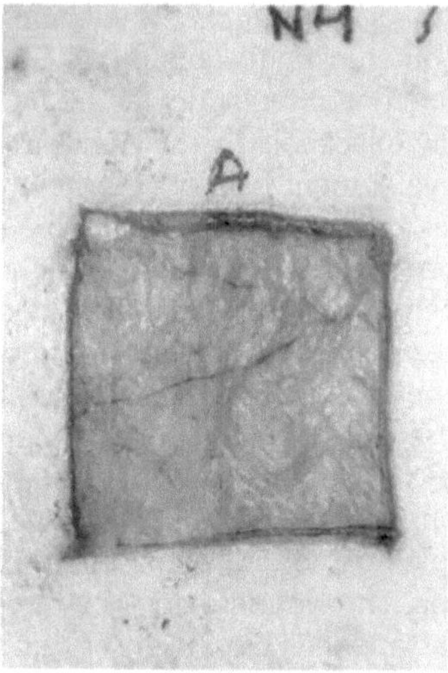

fentanyl i.v.) during the operation, and just before completion and after 8 h 0.005 mg/kg buprenorphine was administered intravenously. During bandage changes the animals were sedated using azaperone 4 mg + atropine 0.5 mg, and then anesthetized using oxygen, nitrous oxide and isoflurane.

Fig. 2. Close-up of an ulcer just before start of treatment

The whole surgical procedure was carried out under sterile conditions. The flank skin was cleansed with cetrimide-chlorhexidine solution 1:30 in alcohol 70%, shaved in the direction of hair growth, rinsed, dried, and then washed with 70% alcohol. An incision of 5 cm length and 2.5 mm depth was made with a scalpel. Starting from this incision the epidermis was excised using the dermatome (Fig 1.). The depth to achieve a full-thickness excision was estimated at 2.4-2.5 mm. The distance between the wounds was 4 cm. To produce a necrotic wound bed the wounds were treated with 20% Trichloroacetic acid. Non-impregnated gauze compresses were applied on the wounds. The wounds were further protected against mechanical trauma with a covering bandage fixed with Me-fix and Tubi-grip.

After 2 days the wounds, covered with a thick layer of necrotic tissue, closely resembled a human necrotic ulcer (Fig 2.) From the third to the tenth day the enzymes and placebo were applied.

Fig. 3. The different products tested in this study

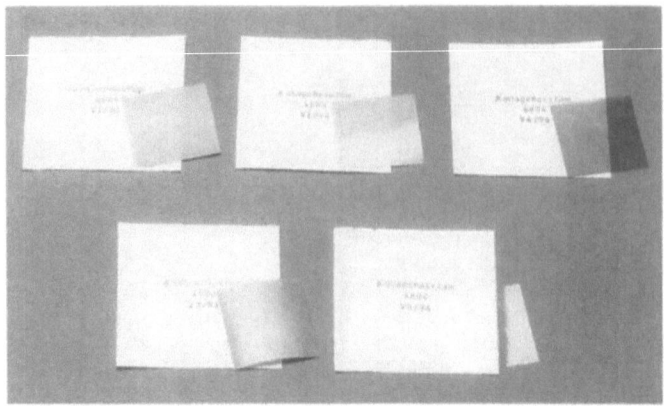

Collagenase Formulations

In this study four dissolvable film sheets containing collagenase in different concentrations (0.5 U/cm^2, 1.0 U/cm^2, 1.0X U/cm^2 (different formulation), and 2.0 U/cm^2) were compared to film only (placebo). The different products are shown in Fig 3. The development goal for the new dosage forms of collagenase was to achieve a fast débridement of necrotic wounds, such as burn wounds. Therefore, a high collagenase concentration is needed, which on the other hand should not harm healthy tissue. Collagenase film is a hydrophillic formulation, which is supposed to dissolve in wound fluid and thus releases the total dose of active ingredient to the wound. Due to the homogenous distribution of collagenase within the film and to the constant thickness of the dosage form, a definite and reproducible dose of collagenase can be applied per cm^2 of wound area. The wounds had to be moist when the study medication was applied. Dry necroses had to be moistened with saline soaked gauzes for 5 minutes until the necrosis was wet. Application to the wounds was accomplished by a person (usually one of the biotechnicians) different from the one who made the clinical observations. The different films and the placebo film were applied once daily for ten days, under occlusion. Clinical evaluation, video photography and computer-aided analysis of wound size and cleanliness were performed daily.

Clinical Observations

The wound size was measured in cm^2 by tracing the wound margins on the screen with a mouse, followed by computerized calculation of the wound surface. Around all wounds a 6 x 6 cm raster was positioned for calibration. Based on the amount of necrotic tissue, slough and granulation tissue in the wound, a visual cleanliness ranking score was given to each wound (1 beeing the cleanest wound). The amount of necrotic tissue, slough and granulation tissue in the wound were estimated visually in percentages by experienced clinical observers (observers were blinded). The number of treatment days necessary to achieve a clean, red, granulating wound bed ('ready for grafting' according to the investigator, which means 95-100% clean) were recorded. Each wound was photographed in color (Polaroids) at regular intervals.

Computer Image Analysis

The débriding effect is usually quantified using the black-yellow-red model, in which black is black necrosis, yellow is yellow necrosis (slough), and red is granulation tissue [2]. This model has been generally accepted by clinicians as a tool to classify wounds on the basis of color. Some pharmaceutical companies have grouped their wound care products according to the same classification model. This three-color visual evaluation model has been used in most clinical trials on wound débridement until now. The computer system is based on the same classification principle. One should realize of course that there are thousands of different hues of red in granulation tissue and that the color of necrotic tissue varies from white, yellow, greenish, hemorrhagic brown to deep black, including all colors in between.

Recording Procedure

A video image of the wounds was obtained by positioning a video camera and a light source, both mounted with polaroid

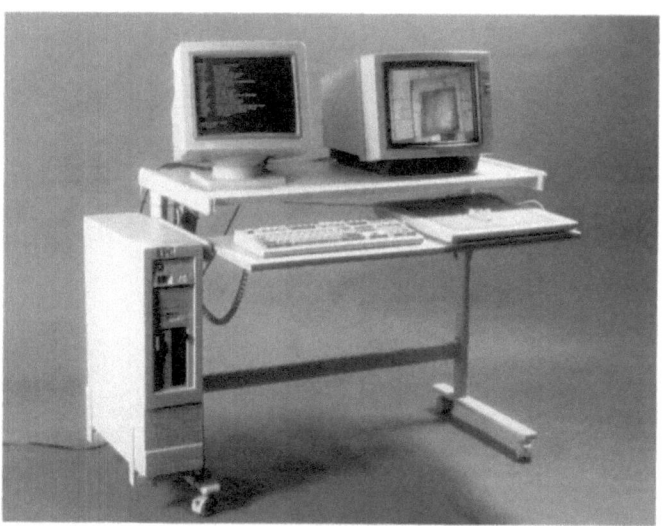

Fig. 4. The computer image analysis system: an IBM-compatible personal computer, a frame grabber, a VGA monitor and an RGB monitor, and a digitizing tablet

filters to prevent reflection, in a standardized way to the wound. All variables such as height, distance, angle, light, diaphragm, etc. were recorded. A color scale and grey scale were positioned near the wounds for calibration purposes.

Hardware

The computer system consists of an IBM-compatible personal computer, a frame grabber, a VGA monitor and an RGB monitor, and a digitizing tablet (Fig 4). Since each stored image requires 500 Kb, two large hard disks and a tape streamer were installed.

Software

The software was specially written by the Department of Medical Physics of the Academical Medical Center, University of Amsterdam, and consists of a mixture of the original software provided with the frame grabber (VISION), programs written in the language C, and a menu structure composed of MS-DOS batch files.

Measurement Procedures

After restoring the image from disk or tape, the ulcer outline was traced on the screen, using the digitizing tablet. Three orientation points around the wound were clicked on with the mouse. After entering the previously recorded horizontal and vertical distances between these orientation marks into the computer, the red, yellow, black, and total wound areas were

Fig. 5. a Image of an animal wound, photographed directly from the computer monitor. The red granulating wound area is clearly distinguishable but, because of the complex two-dimensional structure, difficult to estimate. **b** Recognition of the different areas by the computer system (red is granulation tissue, yellow is necrotic tissue)

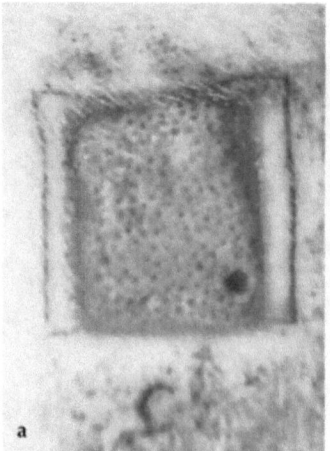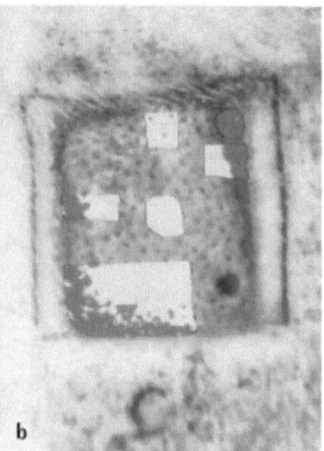

a   b

calculated, in pixels, percentages, and square millimetres. It took about 2 min to fully measure one wound. Figure 5a, photographed directly from the computer monitor, shows an animal wound. The red granulating wound area is clearly distinguishable, but because of the complex two-dimensional structure difficult to estimate. Figure 5b shows how the areas were recognized by the computer system.

Primary Outcome Parameters

The primary measurement of efficacy was wound cleanliness after one week as determined by digital image analysis. Wound cleanliness was assessed electronically using three measurements: necrotic tissue, slough, and granulation tissue. The area of the wound containing necrotic tissue, slough, and granulation tissue each was recorded in mm^2, as a percentage of the total wound area, and as a percentage of the total wound area of the first day (differences were described as change from baseline). Only the computer measurements were used in the data analysis. Student's T-test was used for statistical analysis.

Wound size was not an important parameter in this study. The primary parameter is wound cleaning, not wound healing. The observation period of 10 days is too short to accomplish complete healing. The wound size can be expected to decrease slightly in area as healing occurs. This decrease is greatly caused by wound contraction. The rate of wound contraction is different in different regions on the back, but the randomization will counteract this confounding process. In the first 2-3 days wounds may become bigger because of hydration of the wound bed and the disturbance of the skin integrity by cutting 2.5 mm deep.

Results

The amount of necrotic tissue in each wound was measured in square mm using digital image analysis. This surface was divided by the total wound size before treatment. The result is a percentage of the original wound surface at day 0. So at day 1 there is 100% necrosis, at day 3 usually slightly more than 100% due to hydrolysis of the wound, and then the percentages diminish. At the end, usually around day 10-14, all wounds are clean or nearly clean, but there is a difference in the speed of cleaning. The largest differences can be observed between day 5-8. During treatment the total wound size diminishes, due to epithelialization from the margins and con-

Fig. 6. Amount of necrotic tissue present in the wound after 1 week of treatment with 4 new experimental film formulations of collagenase, in concentrations ranging from 0.5 to 2 units/cm², and a placebo film. The error bars indicate the 95% confidence intervals

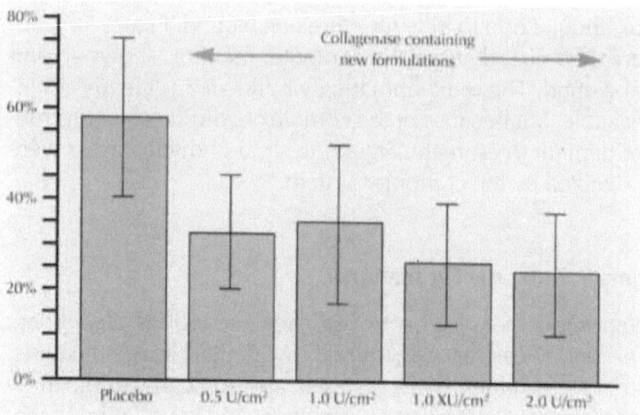

Table 1. Statistical significance (p-values) of the differences between collagenase film and placebo film (Student's t-test)

	Collagenase concentration:			
	0.5 U	1.0 U	1.0XU	2.0 U
Day 6	0.031	0.040	0.013	0.052
Day 7	0.016	0.040	0.003	0.002
Day 8	0.013	n.s.	0.004	0.026

n.s. Not significant at a P-level of 0.05.

traction. The results obtained with the collagenase films are shown in Fig 6. All films containing collagenase were significantly ($p < 0.05$) better than placebo and there was a dose-dependent effect (see Table 1).

Discussion

For a good interpretation of the results one should realize that removal of necrotic tissue during treatment does not instantly reveal granulation tissue, but it allows for the formation of granulation tissue. Once granulation tissue has been formed near the margin of an ulcer, it will be overgrown with epithelium. As a result, the total wound size will be reduced. This means that the relative amount of granulation tissue first increases, but then diminishes. Therefore, the best method for evaluating débridement is to measure the surface covered with necrotic tissue in square millimeters. During the first days of treatment the total wound size may increase as a result of the moisturizing effect of most débriding products.

The collagenase films were all clearly better than the placebo film. The differences were significant. The 2.0 U/cm^2 and the 1.0X U/cm^2 were more effective than the 0.5 U films, but this difference was not significant. Because all films were significantly better than placebo film, the conclusion can be drawn that this formulation might be successful in practice.

The computer image analysis procedure is according to our knowledge the most objective and most appropriate evaluation method for these kind of wounds. Because the wounds are not too deep and not on a convex surface, sharp close-up video-images can be obtained. The advantage of the video system is that the quality (focus, brightness, color saturation) of the stored images can be checked immediately. The high standardization of all variables, especially the light conditions during recording, makes it possible for one single classification table to be used for all animals.

In this study, different concentrations of collagenase in dry film-formulations were used. Because these films need some fluid to dissolve, all wounds had to be moisturized for some minutes. As a consequence, these film formulations may be less suitable to treat dried-out necrotic tissue and dry eschars. This is a question for further research.

References

1. Haury B, Rodeheaver G, Vensko J (1978) Debridement: an essential component of traumatic wound care. Amer J Surg; 135:238-242.
2. Stotts NA (1990) Seeing red, yellow and black. The three-color concept of wound care. Nursing; 20:59-61.
3. Perednia D (1991) What dermatologists should know about digital imaging. J Amer Acad Dermatol ;25:89-108.
4. Smith DJ, Bhat S, Bulgrin JP (1992) Video image analysis of wound repair. Wounds; 4:6-15.
5. Engström N, Hansson F, Hellgren L, Johansson T, Nordin B, Vincent J, Wahlberg A (1990) Computerized wound image analysis. In: Pathogenesis of wound and biomaterial-associated infections. (Eds) T. Wadstrom, I. Eliasson, I. Holder and A. Ljungh, pp 189-192. Springer-Verlag London
6. van Riet Paap E, Mekkes JR, Estevez O, Westerhof W (1991) A new color video image analysis system for the objective assessment of wound healing in secondary healing ulcers. Wounds; 3:47.
7. Westerhof W (ed) (1993) Leg ulcers: diagnosis and treatment. Elsevier, Amsterdam.
8. Mekkes JR, Westerhof W, van Riet Paap E, Habraken J, Estevez O (1994) Evaluation of wound debridement using computerized image analysis. In: Westerhof W, Vanscheidt W. (eds). Proteolytic enzymes and wound healing. Heidelberg, Springer Verlag.
9. Mekkes JR, Westerhof W (1995) Image processing in the study of wound healing. Clinics in Dermatology; 13:401-407
10. Meyer W, Schwarz R, Neurand K (1970) The skin of domestic mammals as a model for the human skin, with special reference to the domestic pig. Curr Probl Dermatol, vol 7, pp. 39-52. Karger, Basel.

Interview

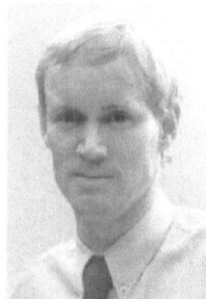

The influence of the vehiculum on wound healing is a very neglected field of research. Can you tell us some preliminary results of your ongoing study?

Mekkes: The excipient of wound-care products is as important as the active ingredients it should contain, conserve, and release to the wound bed. For some wounds it should be dry and absorbing; for other wounds it should provide a humid environment. The excipient itself may be effective apart from the ingredients. The contribution of the separate components can be analysed in our wound model. In this study all new galenic formulations of collagenase were significantly better than the excipient alone, and the effect was dose dependent.

How did the enzyme preparations compare with saline-soaked gauzes in your study?

Mekkes: Saline-soaked gauzes, applied under plastic occlusion as in this study, should not be considered a placebo but rather an accepted control treatment. Despite this fact, the collagenase preparations were superior to saline-soaked gauzes, and the difference was statistically significant.

Was there any difference between saline-soaked gauzes and placebo in your study?

Mekkes: As expected, saline-soaked gauzes were clearly more effective than placebo, but the difference was not significant because of the relatively small sample size (ten wounds in each treatment group).

Enzymatic Débridement of Burn Wounds

J. F. Hansbrough and W. Hansbrough

Summary

Principles for the use of exogenous enzymes as débriding agents for burn wounds are briefly discussed. These agents may be utilized in an attempt to accelerate the removal of devitalized tissue from the wound, and this action will hopefully promote wound closure. Past experience has demonstrated that partial-thickness burn wounds which close quickly heal with less hypertrophic scar than wounds which close more slowly. Since 75% of the dry weight of skin is composed of collagen, exogenous collagenase preparations may prove useful for the débridement of burn wounds. We describe a recent clinical study of the use of a collagenase derived from the bacterium *Clostridium histolyticum*. Seventy-six patients were studied at seven different United States burn centers. Paired partial-thickness wounds in each patient were treated with silver sulfadiazine or collagenase ointment. The use of collagenase ointment resulted in more rapid removal of debris from the wound surface and more rapid epithelialization of the wounds compared with silver sulfadiazine, with statistical significance achieved for both end points ($P < 0.001$). In addition, wounds treated with collagenase ointment were not found to produce more discomfort than wounds treated with silver sulfadiazine, and infection incidences were not different. After completion of the multicenter study, we actively examined the use of collagenase ointment for treating other types of wounds in burn patients, including infected donor sites and chronic, slowly healing partial-thickness burns, and have found it efficacious. Continued study of enzymatic débriding agents for wounds in burn patients will hopefully delineate techniques which will encourage wound closure while simultaneously decreasing the intensity and expense of wound care.

Regional Burn Center, U.S.C.D. Medical Center, 200 West Arbor Drive, San Diego, CA 92103-8896, USA

Clinical Review of Enzymatic Débridement

The goals of local burn wound treatment are to protect against infection and trauma as we care for the wound. We would like to accelerate the removal of devitalized tissue, if that is possible, while utilizing treatment methods which promote rapid wound healing and wound closure. In general, we have learned that partial-thickness burn wounds which close (i.e., epithelialize) quickly heal with less hypertrophic scar than wounds which close more slowly [1, 2]. Therefore, there may be a lasting advantage to the patient when the rapidity of wound healing is accelerated, as well as the potential for lower treatment costs.

The most common methodology for treating partial-thickness burns in the U.S., and probably throughout the world, involves the use of topical antimicrobial agents. The most commonly utilized topical agent in the United States is silver sulfadiazine (SSD). This drug was developed in the 1960s [3, 4]; it is effective for controlling microbial growth in the burn wound as the eschar separates and epithelialization can proceed, resulting in ultimate wound closure. However, the SSD molecule is hydrophobic and, possibly for this reason, application of the topical cream induces the accumulation of significant amounts of proteinaceous exudates on the wound surface. These exudates are commonly termed pseudoeschar, and efforts must be made to gradually remove this tenacious layer of material from the wound surface or bacterial colonization of the wound may progress, resulting in infection and delayed wound healing. Although there has been some suspicion that SSD may actually retard wound healing, there is no clear clinical evidence for this effect.

Although the rather standardized topical method of treating burns is effective, there are considerations which deserve attention. The use of SSD on partial-thickness burns requires the accompanying use of mechanical débriding action, to remove eschar and accumulating proteinaceous debris. The débriding process must be vigorous, if substantial amounts of debris are to be removed from the wound, and simply placing the patient in a whirlpool bath is not effective. Assistance in promoting the removal of necrotic debris is necessary to permit the wound to heal, since the process of epithelialization must proceed across a clean wound bed which is free of debris. Unfortunately, the débriding process may be extremely painful and stressful for the patient and may require the use of heavy doses of analgesics. Extensive wound débridements also may require large time commitment from the nursing staff. It may be difficult for the patient, family, and support staff to accomplish thorough wound cleaning on an outpatient basis, largely because of the high degree of discomfort associated with local wound treatment. Inadequate débridement of the burn wound will lead to persistence of necrotic debris, which conceals the wounds from view, prevents the ongoing evaluation of healing, and may promote infection from growth of micro-organisms in the necrotic tissue and accumulating wound secretions.

Endogenous proteases are secreted by various cells in the wound; these enzymes promote the liquefaction and removal of necrotic tissue and pseudoeschar so that wound healing can proceed. In fact, wound healing requires carefully regulated, spatially organized degradation of collagen [5]. In the case of partial-thickness burn wounds, devitalized proteinaceous debris must be removed to permit epithelial cells to be able to migrate and resurface the wound. Nature has provided an extremely effective method for achieving removal of collagen from wounds; as needed, cells produce enzymes (collagenases) which act primarily, if not exclusively, on collagen [5, 6]. Collagenases work at physiologic pH and temperature. The action of collagenases results in rapid solubilization and denaturation of insoluble native collagen, at which point the proteins are degradable by any number of less specific proteases which may be present in tissues and wounds. While fibroblasts are primary producers, keratinocytes [7] and inflammatory cells [8] can also produce collagenase.

Endogenous collagenases therefore perform an important function in clearing wounds of proteinaceous debris. While various exogenous protease preparations have been utilized for several decades to hasten the débridement process in burn wounds, with the aim of providing great increases in the rate of local protein degradation [9], until the past several years, no controlled trials of enzymatic débriding agents for partial-thickness burn wounds which are permitted to spontaneously heal have been reported in the literature. Accelerated débridement of devitalized tissues and denatured protein would be expected to speed the clearance of eschar and debris from the wound surface. Hopefully, wound healing will be hastened, since the process of epithelialization can proceed unencumbered across the clean wound surface. This may translate to shortened hospitalization times, lower intensity and fewer hours of local wound care, and less patient discomfort. These considerations led to the development of a controlled, randomized prospective trial of collagenase/polymyxin B sulfate/bacitracin powder versus the topical antimicrobial agent silver sulfadiazine for the treatment of partial-thickness burn wounds, which will be discussed here.

There are some potential advantages to using exogenous enzymatic débriding agents on partial-thickness burn wounds. We hope to hasten the removal of the eschar and pseudoeschar which forms. In addition, we may be able to facilitate the evaluation of wound depth, since the wounds may be covered by a thick layer of devitalized dermis and epidermis, as well as by wound secretions. It may take several days and even several weeks, as we follow the wounds, to determine if they will close by epithelialization.

There are also potential disadvantages accompanying the use of enzymatic débriding agents. Enzymes have no inherent antimicrobial activity, and the peptide products of enzymatic digestion may facilitate microbial growth in the wound and thus potentiate infections. There are also reports that enzymatic débriding agents may produce discomfort as they remove necrotic tissue and debris. We need to address these characteristics of any débriding agent which we utilize and make sure it is compatible with our clinical use.

There are several enzymatic débriding agents which are utilized today. Most of them have non specific proteolytic activity but are less effective than collagenase in digesting collagen. Approximately 75% of the dry weight of skin is made up of collagen, so it does make sense to have an active collagenase for maximizing wound débridement.

An enzymatic agent which has been available for many years and which has undergone active study in the past several years for burns is collagenase ointment, which is distributed by Knoll Pharmaceutical Company. This enzyme preparation, derived from the bacterium *Clostridium histolyticum,* digests necrotic collagen. Although collagenase ointment was approved for débriding wounds, including burns, approximately 20 years ago, there has been no systematic controlled study of its use in burns until the past several years.

Dr. Harry Soroff completed and published a pilot study in which he treated 13 burn patients with collagenase ointment and silver sulfadiazine on paired, comparison wound sites [10]. Patients with two matching deep dermal burns were chosen to determine the comparative effects of the two agents on wound cleaning and wound healing. To summarize his findings, the first end point evaluated was the number of days until a clean wound bed was achieved. This was defined as the number of days until injured dermis and debris were removed. Dr. Soroff found that in the 13 patients the median number of days to a clean wound bed in collagenase-treated wound sites was 6 days, compared with 12 days in control sites treated with silver sulfadiazine ($P = 0.0012$). Wounds were treated until complete epithelialization occurred. Dr. Soroff found more rapid epithelialization in wound sites treated with collagenase ointment, with a mean of 10 days versus 15 days in the silver sulfadiazine-treated sites ($P = 0.0007$).

Multicenter Evaluation of Collagenase Treatment of Burn Wounds

Following evaluation of the small pilot study by Dr. Soroff, Knoll Pharmaceutical Company decided to proceed into a multicenter study to further study the effects of collagenase ointment on burn wounds [11]. This was a carefully designed, randomized prospective study which required paired burn sites in each patient. These wounds consisted of two partial-thickness burns which were judged by the clinicians to be of comparable area and depth. Choosing such matching wound sites is not particularly easy, and the accrual rate was slow because the investigators were very careful in choosing paired wounds of equivalent depth which were anatomically separate. Once the patients were entered into the study, the wounds were randomly assigned to receive either collagenase ointment plus polymyxin B sulfate/bacitracin powder or silver sulfadiazine. Although the polymyxin B sulfate/bacitracin antimicrobial agent is not actively absorbed into the tissues, it was utilized to achieve some measure of antimicrobial activity in the dissolving tissues. Preliminary studies by Knoll Pharmaceuticals Inc. demonstrated that polymyxin B sulfate/bacitracin powder did not decrease the enzymatic activity of collagenase.

The topical treatments were begun within 4 days of burn inury. We believe that early treatment is important because past experience shows that after several days to a week the eschar can desiccate and become very resistant to any type of enzymatic débridement. We continued topical treatment at each site with the two agents until the site was determined to be clean of debris and the wound could be placed into a semi-occlusive dressing.

There were two end points in this study. The first was the number of days until a clean wound bed was achieved, free of superficial debris, which permitted the use of a semi-occlusive dressing. The second was the number of days until complete healing of the wound was achieved by epithalialization. There were seven different investigator groups which contributed patients to the study; a total of 79 patients were enrolled, and

Fig. 1. Partial-thickness burn wound on the arm, 6 days following initiation of treatment with collagenase ointment. The wound is free of necrotic dermis and debris and is ready for placement into a semi-occlusive dressing

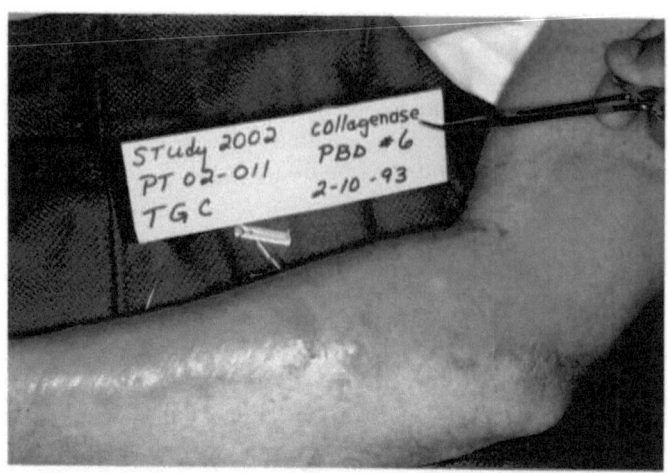

Fig. 2. Burn wound of similar depth on the opposite arm of the same patient, treated with silver sulfadiazine. Significant necrotic material remains on day 6 of treatment; the wound is not ready for application of an occlusive dressing

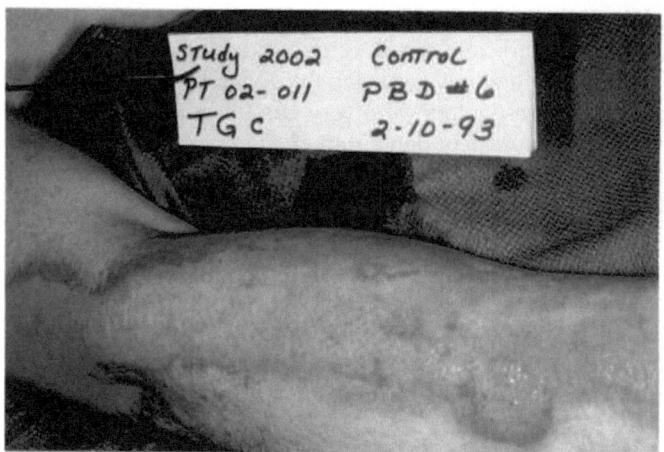

76 were evaluable. The mean burn size was 14% TBSA; the mean patient age was 34 years. The study sites averaged approximately 2% body surface area, since we wanted to be conservative and study relatively modest-sized burn sites until we were confident that we would not have a problem with infections. The collagenase-treated sites and the silver sulfadiazine-treated sites were very comparable in size.

We chose patients for this study who had paired wounds which we felt would probably heal within 7 days to 2–3 weeks. This is always a judgement call for the clinician, and we know that sometimes we are wrong and the wounds fail to heal. In fact, a certain number of wounds failed to heal and required skin grafting, indicating that these particular wounds were not superficial.

Figures 1 and 2 show burns on one of our patients who was admitted with very similar depth wounds on the arms from a flash-flame injury. On day 6 post injury, the collagenase-treated site is free of necrotic debris and is ready for placement into semi-occlusive dressing. The silver sulfadiazine-treated site still contains surface debris; it was not ready for application of a semi-occlusive dressing until day 10 of treatment. The collagenase-treated site was epithelialized on day 8 of treatment, while the silver sulfadiazine site was not healed until day 17.

When we summarized the data on all 76 evaluable patients, the sites treated with collagenase cleaned in less time (mean 9.3 days) than the control sites treated with silver sulfadiazine (mean 11.6 days). This 2.3-day difference was statistically significant ($P = 0.001$) using Student's t-test.

When numbers of days to healed wound were compared, the collagenase-treated sites healed faster than the control sites treated with silver sulfadiazine (mean 19.0 versus 22.1 days). This 3.1-day difference was statistically significant ($P = 0.001$).

The hallmark of any study in which deep partial-thickness wounds are evaluated which the clinician believes will heal in 2–3 weeks is that some of the wounds will fail to heal and will require excision and grafting. Indeed, this did occur in some patients. Fourteen collagenase-treated sites and 18 sites treated with silver sulfadiazine required excision and grafting (nonsignificant). There was also no difference between the two groups in terms of numbers of wounds which developed mild infections.

The general impressions of our clinicians, the research nurses, and also our staff burn nurses who cared for these patients were that the silver sulfadiazine-treated sites were more painful during the débriding process compared with the collagenase-treated sites. It appeared that there was less effort involved in cleaning up the collagenase-treated sites, and that the debris in the wound was much easier to remove since it was partially digested.

After evaluating the first dozen patients at our site, we decided to investigate the levels of discomfort more objectively, in a prospective fashion, to determine if there indeed was a difference in discomfort between the two treatment methods. We utilized the standard visual analog scale in the subsequent 19 patients at our Burn Center who were enrolled in the clinical study. Pain was measured at three time points on each day of treatment: during débridement, 15 min after débridement, and

Fig. 3 a–c. Patient-generated pain scores (10-point visual analog scale) are shown for each day of treatment in a subset of 19 patients. Patients were requested to estimate their pain during débridement (**a**), 15 min following débridement (**b**), and 30 min following débridement (**c**). A higher score indicates greater discomfort reported by the patient. Pain was less in almost all patients in wounds treated with collagenase ointment compared with silver sulfadiazine-treated wounds

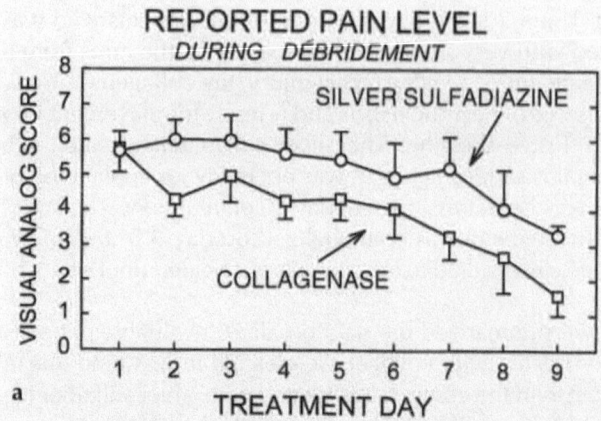

REPORTED PAIN LEVEL
DURING DÉBRIDEMENT

SILVER SULFADIAZINE

COLLAGENASE

VISUAL ANALOG SCORE

TREATMENT DAY

a

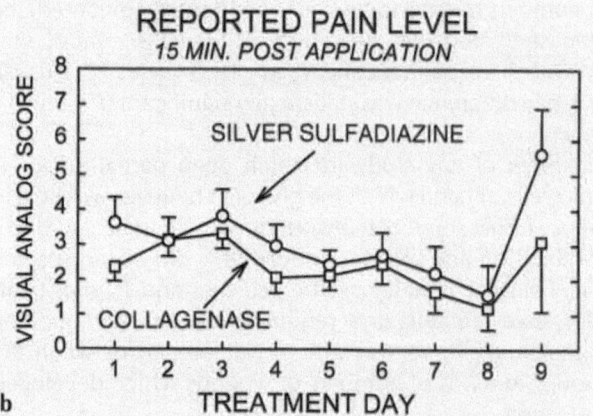

REPORTED PAIN LEVEL
15 MIN. POST APPLICATION

SILVER SULFADIAZINE

COLLAGENASE

VISUAL ANALOG SCORE

TREATMENT DAY

b

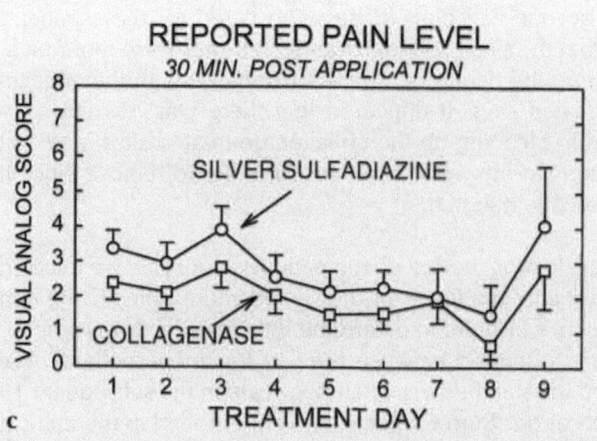

REPORTED PAIN LEVEL
30 MIN. POST APPLICATION

SILVER SULFADIAZINE

COLLAGENASE

VISUAL ANALOG SCORE

TREATMENT DAY

c

30 min after débridement. The patient pointed to a mark way to the left of the scale if he or she felt there was no pain, and to a mark way to the right of the scale if the pain was perceived as being the worst imaginable. The demographic characteristics of this subset of 19 patients were similar to those of the total patient group.

Figure 3 shows the results of the measures of discomfort in the 19 patients during débridement. Again, higher scores indicate increasing levels of discomfort. Upon examining mean scores for each treatment day up to 9 days it can be seen that on essentially each day of treatment the numerical pain score is less in the collagenase-treated group. Because there are only 19 patients, statistical differences were found only at several days of evaluation. Clearly, however, there was not an increase in pain during the débriding process in patients treated with collagenase ointment throughout the treatment period. At 15 and 30 min following débridement and reapplication of either collagenase or silver sulfadiazine, we again found no increased discomfort in the collagenase-treated sites.

Collagenase for Débriding Other Wounds

After completion of the multicenter study, we actively investigated the use of collagenase ointment for treating a variety of wounds in our burn patients. Donor sites pose a particular problem in burn patients. These wounds frequently become infected and develop accumulated drainage and debris, and they often produce more discomfort and associated anxiety for the patient than the actual burn wounds.

Collagenase ointment has proven very effective for "cleaning up" these wounds. These wounds frequently develop problems 5–7 days postoperatively, including the accumulation of proteinaceous debris which clings to the wound. Enzymatic treatment for several days promotes débridement of the wounds, permitting the early application of a semi-occlusive dressing which can be left in place until epithelialization proceeds and closes the wound.

Pressure ulcers, venous ulcers, and other types of chronic wounds have been treated with collagenase ointment for the past several decades, and the enzyme functions very effectively in this regard. Our Burn Center includes a busy outpatient wound care center, and many patients with wound problems are treated with collagenase ointment for various periods of time to "clean up" their wounds. The results are generally excellent, as exemplified by the avulsion injury in a steroid-treated patient shown in Fig. 4.

Fig. 4 a–c. Chronic wounds on a patient who suffered an avulsion injury to the arm. The patient was on high-dose corticosteroids following lung transplantation, and the wound showed a thick layer of debris *(a)*. **b** Following 10 days' treatment with collagenase ointment, the wounds were free of debris and could be treated with an occlusive dressing. **c** The wounds then closed nicely

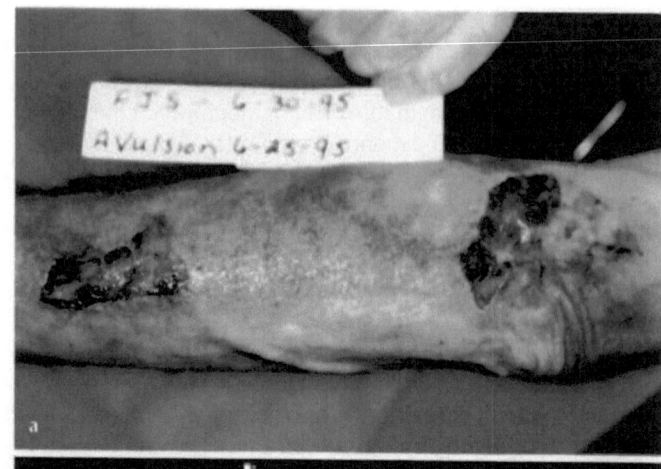

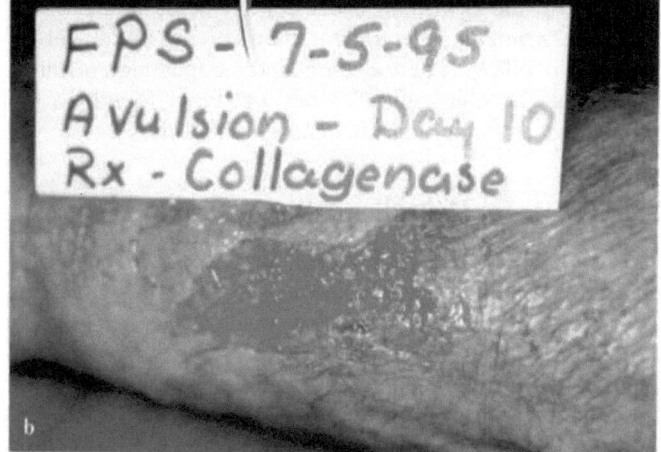

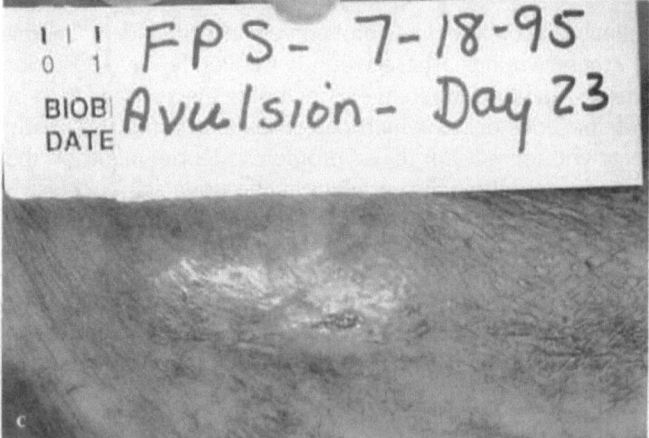

Table 1. Comparison of collagenase and silver sulfadiazine on partial-thickness burn wounds

	Colla-genase	SSD	Difference	P value[a]
Days to clean wound				
No. of patients	76	76		
Mean (days)	9.3	11.6	−2.3	0.001
Median (days)	7	9		
Days to healed wound				
No. of patients	76	76		
Mean (days)	19	22.1	−3.1	0.001
Median (days)	15	18		

[a] Mean days were compared using Students' τ-test.
SSD, silver sulfadiazine

Conclusions

Although enzymatic débriding agents may be valuable adjuncts in burn wound care, there have been few carefully controlled studies of their use. We believe that collagenase treatment in patients with moderate-extent partial-thickness burns results in less discomfort during the débriding process and promotes earlier removal of necrotic debris from the wound. Earlier cleaning of the wound appears to correlate with more rapid epithelialization in the collagenase-treated wound sites. The results of this clinical trial encourage further study of the efficacy of enzymatic agents for treatment of burn wounds. It appears that more widespread use of enzymatic débriding agents such as collagenase ointment can improve the outcomes of burn injuries in selected patients, and these agents may also lower the intensity of wound care and ultimately decrease the costs of burn care.

References

1. Moncrief JA (1979) Topical antibacterial treatment of the burn wound. In: Artz CP, Moncrief JA, Pruitt BA jr (eds) Burns: a team approach. Saunders, Philadelphia, pp 250–269
2. Deitch EA, Wheelahan TM, Rose MP, et al (1983) Hypertrophic burn scars: analysis of variables. J Trauma 23 : 895–898
3. Moncrief JA, Lindberg RB, Switzer WE, Pruitt BA jr (1966) Use of tropical antibacterial therapy in the treatment of the burn wound. Arch Surg 92 : 558–565
4. Fox CL jr (1969) Clinical experience with silver sulfadiazine: a new topical agent for control of *Pseudomonas* infections in burns. J Trauma 9 : 377-388

5. Jeffrey JJ (1992) Collagen degradation. In: Cohen IK, Diegelmann RF, Lindblad WJ (eds) Wound healing: biochemical and clinical aspects. Saunders, Philadelphia, pp 177–194
6. Eisen AZ, Jeffrey JJ, Gross J (1968) Human skin collagenase. Isolation and mechanism of attack on the collagen molecule. Biochim Biophys Acta 161 : 637–645
7. Peterson MJ, Woodley DT, Stricklin GP, O'Keefe EJ (1987) Production of procollagenase by cultured human keratinocytes. J Biol Chem 262 : 835–840
8. Wahl LM, Wahl SM, Mergenhagen S, Martin GR (1975) Collagenase production by lymphokine-activated macrophages. Science 187 : 261–263
9. Silverstein P, Maxwell PJ, Duckett L (1987) Enzymatic débridement. In: Bowsick J (ed) The art and science of burn care. Aspen, Rockville., pp 75–81
10. Soroff HS, Sasvary DH (1994) Collagenase ointment and polymyxin B sulfate/bacitracin spray versus silver sulfadiazine cream in partial thickness burns: a pilot study. J Burn Care Rehab 15 : 13–17
11. Hansbrough JF, Achauer B, Dawson J, et al (1995) Wound healing in partial-thickness burn wounds treated with collagenase ointment versus silver sulfadiazine cream. J Burn Care Rehab 16 : 241–247

Interview

What is the main conclusion you draw from this multicenter study for practical work in burn care?

Hansbrough: Collagenase ointment has been shown in extensive, controlled clinical studies to result in accelerated débriding and healing of limited-surface-area, partial-thickness burn wounds (up to approximately 15% of the body surface area). In addition, patients report less discomfort during and after the débriding process, apparently because the enzyme helps to digest the necrotic debris on the wound surface, which makes it easier for the nurses to clean the wound during the dressing change/débridement procedure. This agent can be a valuable adjunct in the treatment of burn wounds.

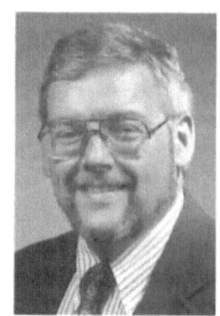

Is it still justified to use only topical antibiotics in the treatment of burn wounds?

Hansbrough: There are several different ways in which to treat burn wounds. When the wounds cover extensive areas of the body, and the risk of generalized wound sepsis is present, most areas of the wounds are probably best treated with topical antimicrobial agents to control bacterial proliferation. Our studies demonstrate that partial-thickness burn wounds of limited to moderate surface area, covering up to 15% of the body surface area, can be safely treated with collagenase ointment, combined with the use of polymyxin B sulfate/bacitracin powder to achieve some level of antimicrobial action in the liquifying eschar.

Which studies are still needed for a future decision tree for burn wound care?

Hansbrough: It would be very helpful to study the use of more concentrated preparations of the collagenase, to determine if eschar removal can be accelerated even further with the continued avoidance of discomfort. In addition, combined use of collagenase ointment with effective topical antimicrobial agents, such as silver sulfadiazine, should be investigated for the treatment of burn wounds covering larger areas.

Subject Index